CW01090917

AGEING GRACEFULLY

AGEING GRACEFULLY

A Holistic Guide to Later Life

Elisabeth Brooke

AEON

First published in 2024 by
Aeon Books

British Library Cataloguing in Publication Data

A C.I.P. for this book is available from the British Library

ISBN-13: 978-1-80152-102-4

Typeset by Medlar Publishing Solutions Pvt Ltd, India

www.aeonbooks.co.uk

CONTENTS

INTRODUCTION

The idea for writing this book was to investigate ageing as I am approaching my 70th year. Having been involved in natural medicine all my adult life, my health is good, but how could I ensure it stayed that way? I am sure we all have a dread of ending up as that person drooling in a chair, staring vacantly and unknowingly out into a room full of similar empty bodies. I wanted to investigate how I could minimise the risk of that happening to me.

It has been a fascinating journey looking at the latest research into ageing, there is loads, and investigating other things like happiness, fun, and kindness as well as the more predictable diet, lifestyle, etc.

The book is divided into two parts. Part I looks at the fundamentals of staying healthy. These apply to any age but are especially important because as we grow older, our bodies can become less resilient and the effects of a lifetime's habits may begin to show up in the body.

Chapter 1, Nourishment, talks about food, eating habits, and staying healthy. Some of the ideas I discuss may surprise, while others will be more familiar. I start with nourishment as the food we eat is the building block of both health and disease. The choice is ours. Changing your diet at any age can have dramatic results; it really is never too late to change.

The second chapter is Rest. Sleep can become an issue as we age, so in this chapter I talk about the importance of sleep in our bodies, and how sleep is an active state where the body repairs itself and prepares our brain for the next day. There is lots we can do to achieve a good, restful sleep.

Chapter 3, Stretch, discusses the importance of exercise as we grow older. Our bodies are designed to move, and move we must if we wish to stay healthy, bright, and happy. Exercise doesn't have to be the sweaty experience we had when we were younger; there are lots of ways to get moving that are pleasurable.

Chapter 4, Thinking, discusses the science (as we know it to date) of the brain. Dementia is a big issue as we age, but there are many things we can do to keep our minds well-exercised and healthy.

I discuss Happiness in Chapter 5. Happiness is one of the major factors which determine how we age, our longevity, and health. As we grow older, our moods may dip as we lose loved ones, retire, or feel our life has changed in ways we cannot control. Cultivating happiness is an art we can all practice.

Chapter 6 is Connection. Our social relationships are a major factor in healthy old age. Indeed, research among the most long-lived populations showed that having a close-knit group around you brings extraordinary benefits. Our society has become more solitary, and we may well have lost friends and family members and experience, perhaps for the first time, loneliness and isolation. As we age, our interests change; this gives us an opportunity to make new connections and prioritise socialising as well as starting those things 'we always meant to do'.

Chapter 7, Fun, discusses things we can do for pleasure. Fun is very important as we grow older, but our sense of what fun is, of course, changes. There was a meme I saw that sums this up, 'when we were teenagers, we snuck out of the house to go to parties. When we get older, we sneak out of parties to go home'. This chapter looks at ways to have fun and why pleasure keeps us healthy and happy.

Chapter 8, 'Checking out', discusses death and dying. Life, as the cliché goes, is a terminal condition. Death does not have to be a negative experience; it is as natural as birth. In this chapter, I discuss many ways to manage death as a powerful, healing experience rather than a terrifying prospect.

Part II is the practical part of the book, where we can act on what we have learnt in Part I. I have organised it this way as I find it annoying when I can't find some resource mentioned in a chapter without reading all the way through the chapter again.

Part II also contains a herbal Materia Medica, which lists the herbs mentioned and gives some of my favourite recipes for herbal delights. 'Natural quick fixes' go through a number of common conditions, and their remedies.

I hope *Ageing Gracefully* will be an inspiring, informative, and thought-provoking guide to approach our later years.

Fitzrovia, Spring Equinox 2023

PART I

FOUNDATION

CHAPTER 1

Nourishment

How boring! I expect you are waiting for me to tell you what to eat and to lose weight and count calories and stop eating butter and cakes and all the nice things. Well, I might do a little of that, but principally I would like to share with you the current thinking on diet, both mainstream and alternative viewpoints, which is radically different from the common consensus that has been around since the 1990s.

We were told that fats were bad and that a low-carb diet would be the solution to heart disease, type 2 diabetes, obesity, etc. However, after 30 years under this regime, the incidence of hypertension, type 2 diabetes, and cancer has hardly changed, and in many cases has increased exponentially.

If you look to the next page under 'For conspiracy theorists', you will see the background to these beliefs.

Putting things in context, doctors, both here and in the US, are taught virtually nothing about food and diet. The whole emphasis of modern medicine has been towards treatment and not prevention: high blood pressure, take a pill; obesity, have an operation; diabetes, have a pill; and so on. Until fairly recently, there has been little discussion as to *why* people develop these conditions.

It is known that people in more traditional communities, like the Plains Indians, people in Sardinia, and Seventh Day

Adventists (known as the Blue Zone), eat an unprocessed diet, and their health and incidence of cancer, obesity, type 2 diabetes, and hypertension are much lower than those who eat a mainstream diet. Polish women and Japanese women eating a diet high in fermented foods like sauerkraut and miso have a very low incidence of breast cancer. When Japanese and Polish women move to the US, their incidence of breast cancer rises level to that of American women.

So clearly, there is something in the diet which causes these chronic diseases, which are associated with ageing. Some doctors looking for solutions to this conundrum, who call themselves doctors of 'functional medicine',[1] disseminate this research online. Alternative practitioners have long advocated a close examination of diet. Now, there is a multitude of research papers which confirm what complementary practitioners have always known. Good diet heals, bad diet kills.

So, what is a good diet? The groups mentioned above had very different diets; the Plains Indians mainly ate buffalo meat and berries, the Seventh Day Adventists ate a vegetarian diet, and Sardinian shepherds ate vegetables and fish. So, longevity and health in old age do not seem to respond to a particular diet, but what the diets *don't* contain.

The insulin response

Insulin as you probably know is needed to regulate the balance of glucose in the body. But insulin has a far wider effect on all the organs of the body. When we eat something sugary, our insulin levels rise, which causes inflammation throughout the body, including the brain. Continue eating this way and eat more than three times a day. By constant snacking (grazing), the insulin response remains constantly triggered and this does not give the body any 'down time' to recover. As a consequence, the inflammatory state continues and eventually the tissues of the body begin to break down.

How do we reduce the insulin response? You have probably experienced a slump in energy in the afternoons, around 4 pm, and you may also feel tired after a meal. What you are experiencing is a drop in blood glucose. Sometimes you suffer from brain fog, or an urge to eat again. All of these are the insulin response.

You may not always experience these symptoms; check with yourself to see what types of foods make you sleepy, bloated, and irritable.[2] Chances are they are sugary foods and refined carbohydrates like bread, pasta, and highly processed foods (HPFs).

Highly processed foods

HPFs are foods whose ingredients you would not have in your store cupboard and foods whose ingredients you cannot pronounce, for example, disodium inosinate and disodium guanylate (flavour enhancers in pot noodles). Acetic acid, citric acid, sodium citrate (shepherd's pie), E471, soya lecithin, E476 (vegan ice cream). In other words, ingredients which do not occur in nature.

In the last 30 years, the incidence of highly processed foods has risen exponentially and has kept in line with the rise of obesity, type 2 diabetes, and heart disease. Coincidence? No. It is estimated that British teenagers eat 60% of their diet as HPFs, and the incidence of mental health problems and obesity has skyrocketed. Coincidence? No. Besides the weird chemicals, what is it that HPFs contain that appears to be so bad for health? Fructose.

Names for fructose

Corn syrup, high-fructose corn syrup, cane sugar, glucose, agave nectar, dextrose, malt syrup, corn sweetener, ethyl maltol, dextrose, fructose, fruit juice concentrates, invert sugar, lactose, maltose, raw sugar, sucrose, sugar syrup, Florida crystals, barley malt, rice syrup, caramel, panocha, muscovado, molasses, treacle, carob syrup, evaporated cane juice, honey, and turbinado sugar.

Don't think these are just found in sweets and deserts: sugar or fructose is found in all HPFs. Here is an example of ingredients of a high-end supermarket pizza: flavourings: dextrose, sugar; a popular vegetarian sausage: barley malt extract, natural caramelised sugar; while a 'healthy' granola contains: oat flakes, sugar, palm oil, sunflower seeds, coconut, honey (1%) sugar syrup powder, flavouring. Remember, ingredients are listed according to weight, not content, so the heaviest will appear first on the list of ingredients.

What does sugar, particularly in the form of glucose, do to our bodies?

The insulin response

When we eat sugars or refined carbohydrates, the pancreas secretes insulin and this triggers other mechanisms in the body to move the excess sugar to fat stores, which is why if we eat a lot of sugar we get fat.

While insulin is circulating in your bloodstream, after each sugary food, fat is stored, but it cannot be released from fat cells to be used as energy. If you eat sugary or refined carbohydrates every couple of hours, insulin is permanently present in your bloodstream, which means fat is stored but never released from storage to be burned as energy.

The constant presence of insulin in the bloodstream means there are energy slumps as the sugar has been removed from the bloodstream and stored as fat, so the body will crave more sugar to deal with the fluctuating sugar levels in the blood.

Biologically our body has not evolved to deal with huge hits of sugar; refined sugars are a very new addition to our diets.

Eventually, the pancreas adapts, and the body experiences reduced insulin sensitivity. As the body is constantly flooded with sugars and then insulin, it becomes desensitised to sugar, and it takes more and more insulin to remove sugar in the bloodstream. This is how type 2 diabetes develops. As well as many other chronic health conditions; indeed, Alzheimer's has been called type 3 diabetes as it is believed that the constant state of inflammation aggravates the whole body.

Not all carbohydrates are created equal. Vegetables contain fibre which slows the release of the sugars and so don't cause insulin spikes (the exception being potatoes).

The insulin response is implicated in all manner of conditions, from heart disease, obesity, type 2 diabetes, Alzheimer's, and depression.

What does that mean practically?

Prepare food from scratch, or buy food which has been minimally processed; avoid HPFs, takeaways, food which has ingredients not found in an ordinary kitchen, and ingredients you cannot pronounce. Learn to cook simple foods. Get high-quality food; this does not necessarily mean more expense. It has also been found that walking after meals reduces insulin spikes, so consider putting this into your routine.

Benefits

- Healthwise immense.
- Psychologically massive.
- Energy-wise massive.
- Financially, money-saving—HPFs are expensive overall.

So, what to eat?

One of the best ways is to get a food box from a local farmer, which is high in vegetables and fresh as can be. Having paid for them, you are more likely to eat them. The box may seem pricey at first, but when you have most of your food delivered, you no longer go to supermarkets, which means you don't buy things you didn't intend to. We all do this, you go in for one thing and come out with 15, so you will find with the food box you save a lot of money. Don't like all vegetables? You can usually choose your veg for a little extra, so you don't get things you know you won't eat.

Learn to cook.

Even if you have never cooked much, through time pressures or lack of interest or ability, turn cooking once a day into a fun project, or a task to master. You can cook food in batches and freeze portions sizes for those times you can't be bothered to cook, I do this with soups, rice, homemade veggie burgers, sauces for pasta, etc., most things freeze well and if you freeze portions sizes, so they are ready to go.

What you will find

More energy, no more afternoon slump, brain fog will reduce, and many, many symptoms will disappear or lessen in severity. You will lose weight, especially the belly fat, which is where insulin stores all that glucose.

Don't be hardcore.

Unless you have severe symptoms, I recommend that you take a light touch approach and allow yourself little treats from time to time.

Good, dark chocolate, berries, cocoa with nut milks; there are lots of little treats you can have so you don't feel too deprived. Home-cooked treats are always much healthier than shop-bought ones.

Try this diet for a month or six weeks, then have an HPF meal, and see how you feel the next day; that will probably tell you all you need to know about your body and diet. Include your mood, notice if you feel down or irritated or just lazy, and especially notice if you have cravings for more HPFs in subsequent days, as this food is very addictive.

Fats: the good, the bad, and the ugly

Along with the sugar myth came the low-fat myth. Saturated fats are bad (by saturated, I mean animal fats, coconut oils, etc.); polyunsaturated fats (seed oil fats like rapeseed and sunflower oil) are good.

We were told that saturated fats increase cholesterol which causes heart disease and hypertension. Not true. Studies have found no correlation between a high-fat diet and heart disease. The incidence of hypertension has increased, not decreased, since this 'discovery'. What has been found is a correlation between eating seed oils and the insulin response, which we saw above is implicated in heart disease, hypertension, etc.

How are seed oils made? (this includes vegan butters, folks, a popular vegan butter contains sunflower, coconut and rapeseed oils). Seed oils from soya, corn, rapeseed (canola in the US), and sunflower oils have only been in the diet for around 100 years. They were originally developed by Procter and Gamble in the 1870s in the US to make soap, which was previously made from pork fat. Cotton seed oil was thenceforth used in soap making, and it was found that if it was hydrogenated it turned into a solid cooking fat which resembled lard. Soya beans were introduced in the 1930s and soon became the most popular oil. These oils are cheap to produce and entered the processed food market.

The Minnesota Coronary Experiment 1968–1973[3]

In this study, more than 2,300 men and women were randomly assigned to a diet in which all the oils were replaced with vegetable oils, or a control diet high in animal fats. Those who ate more vegetable oils (primarily corn oil) did indeed lower their cholesterol by nearly 14% compared with those who did not, but that after a year or more, they did not see any lower rates of heart disease or dying from heart events. In fact, for every 30 mg/dL drop in cholesterol, there was a 22% increased risk of death. So, cholesterol, although present in heart disease, was seen to be a by-product of the condition, not a cause. Unexpectedly, people who ate animal fats tended to live longer than those who switched to vegetable oils.

The data analysis concluded in 2016 that:

> *No randomized controlled trial has shown that replacement of saturated fat with linoleic acid significantly reduces coronary heart disease events or deaths.*
>
> Conclusions: Available evidence from randomized controlled trials shows that the replacement of saturated fat in the diet with linoleic acid effectively lowers serum cholesterol but does not support the hypothesis that this translates to a lower risk of death from coronary heart disease from all causes. Findings from the Minnesota Coronary Experiment add to growing evidence that incomplete publication has contributed to overestimation of the benefits of replacing saturated fat with vegetable oils rich in linoleic acid.

What this means is that the trial data for cutting out saturated fats from the diet to reduce heart disease failed to publish (or hid) evidence which did not prove their hypothesis. They lied, in other words ...

Saturated fats do not cause heart disease. Vegetable oils lower blood cholesterol, but this has no effect on the rates of coronary heart disease.

Oops ... but what are the effects of seed oils on the body?[4]

Generally, people have taken on board the health advice given in the wake of the Minnesota Study and reduced their intake of saturated fats, salt, reduced smoking, taken more exercise, and eaten more vegetables; yet the rates of chronic disease have skyrocketed. In the US, consumption of vegetable oils has increased five-fold since the mid-1960s, while the incidence of diabetes in that same period has gone from 1.6% of the population to 8.3% in 2020, despite the fact that consumption of sugar and sweeteners (obvious sugars) has flatlined. The same has occurred with smokers: in 1974, 45% of Americans smoked; in 2020, the rate was 13.5%.[5]

Despite this, in the US rates of chronic disease have risen 700% since 1935; 60% of Americans have a chronic disease, while rates of smoking and eating (obvious) sugars have decreased. The consumption of fruit and vegetables and rates of exercise have increased, yet they have had no effect on the rates of chronic disease.[6]

This is counterintuitive. It would be expected that with exercising more and eating healthier (according to medical advice) rates of obesity would be decreasing. The opposite has occurred. In the UK, 28% of adults are obese (2020). In the US, it is 43% (2020). So, what is it that is driving chronic disease and obesity rates? Chronic diseases are seen as ongoing, life-limiting conditions such as diabetes, cancer, heart disease, dementia, obesity, and asthma. In the US, 40% of adults have multiple chronic diseases.

Here is a list of the foods we are eating in the same quantity as 50 years ago:

Animal Fats, eggs, dairy, legumes (beans and pulses), root vegetables, nuts, and fruit. We are also eating similar amounts of sodium (salt), saturated fats, animal foods, cholesterol, fibre, and total carbohydrates.[7] So these cannot account for the rise in chronic disease.

What has increased are these foods:

- Sugar: 88 more calories per day.
- Meat: 125 more calories per day.
- Grains: 185 more calories per day.
- Vegetable oils: 423 more calories per day.[8]

Vegetable oil comprises 20% of the average American diet, and the UK is not far behind.

What effect do vegetable oils have on the body?

The unsaturated fats in seed (vegetable) oils oxidise when they are heated. Oxidation damages tissues and causes inflammation, such as roughening the lining of coronary arteries causing heart attacks. It has been found that these effects are more pronounced over the age of 65, in smokers, and in the presence of other environmental pollutants.[9]

So, not only do seed oils have no effect on mortality from chronic disease, but they can actually cause it by being inflammatory, and the effects are more marked in older people.

So, use good oils like olive oil, coconut oil, lard, butter, and ghee, and avoid foods which are high in vegetable oils. This includes all processed foods and usually restaurant foods and takeaway food, also cheaply produced meat and poultry, which are fed on seed oils.

Digestion

Certainly, our digestion can become weaker as we grow older, and our tolerance for fats, especially, becomes lower. What can be done?

Herbs are great for digestion. A category of remedies known as bitters stimulate the secretion of bile and digestive enzymes, which help to stimulate the whole digestive process. Appetisers and digestives work in the same way|: their bitterness preps the digestive system for food, and coffee; another bitter, traditionally taken after meals, helps in the same way.

Take 10 drops of a tincture, 30 minutes before food or 30 minutes after eating.

My favourites are milk thistle, dandelion root, and agrimony (see Materia Medica).

Sour foods also help digestion and remove trapped wind caused by foods fermenting in the digestive tract.

Cider vinegar is a favourite: 1 tablespoon in a glass of water. All fermented foods have a beneficial effect on the digestive process.

Lemons help to cleanse the system and are an all-round remedy for the gut. If you are using organic or unwaxed lemons, after squeezing them you can use the rind. Cut the rind into strips and soak in water overnight and then strain and drink. It is surprisingly bitter.

Ginger is another helpful digestive remedy. Grate a little (1 inch/2.5 cm) into a glass of water and stand for 30 minutes, then strain and drink. Ginger is especially good for sluggish digestion and bloating, where things need to be speeded up.

Timing

The body loves routine. Try to eat at the same time of day. Eat a large breakfast, a smaller lunch, and a smaller supper. If you are eating healthy foods, you can have large portions. Think about the way people ate in the 1950s, lots of meat and veg and large heavy puddings, yet photographs from that time show very few fat people.

Fasting

Try to leave 12–16 hours between supper and breakfast to give the body time to digest the last meal and heal itself. Space meals out at four-hour intervals. Snacking interferes with digestion, and the insulin response, so avoid eating between meals and snacking before you eat for the same reason.

Constipation

This can be an issue as we age. Do make sure you are drinking enough water, 1–2 litres a day, especially drinking one or two large glasses of water on rising, maybe with a slice of lemon or ginger, is often enough to get things moving. As you begin to eat healthier foods with more roughage, your bowel movements will regularise. Again, try to get into a routine with bowel movements; the body loves the predictable.

CHAPTER 2

Rest

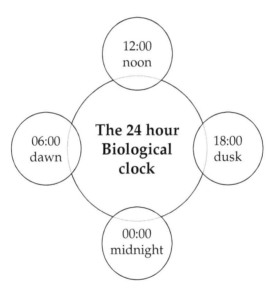

02:00	Deepest sleep	14:30	Best coordination
04:30	Lowest Body Temperature	15:30	Fastest reaction time
06:45	Sharpest rise in blood pressure	17:00	Greatest muscle strength and cardiovascular efficiency
07:30	Melatonin secretion stops	18:30	Highest blood pressure
08:30	Bowel movement likely	19:00	Highest temperature
09:00	Highest testosterone secretion	21:00	Melatonin secretion starts
10:00	High alertness	22.30	Bowel movements suppressed

There is always a reason for insomnia: it is a symptom. Sleep can be a big issue as we grow older, but it doesn't have to be. There are lots of ways we can re-programme our sleep patterns so we can get a restful sleep of seven to nine hours each night.

First, why is it important to get a good night's sleep? Sleep is when our body repairs itself, when our detox system is most active, and when we rest and repair cells throughout the body. It doesn't only relax the whole complex mechanism of our physical body but also rests and replenishes our brain, and our emotions and allows us time to unconsciously process what has happened to us during the day, so that, ideally, we wake up feeling refreshed and ready for a new day.

Hormones are important to consider when we discuss sleep. Seventy per cent of the anti-ageing hormone AGH is produced in the first 70% of sleep time. AGH increases lean body mass and protects bone density and prevents ageing, and promotes brain health. Progesterone is a relaxing hormone which relaxes the body and helps sleep. Falling progesterone levels during menopause can be the reason people who have never had problems sleeping suddenly develop insomnia. Poor absorption can affect progesterone levels in the body (see Nourishment).

Testosterone is found in both men and women. When levels are low, the brain's ability to reset the nervous system is impaired, causing brain fog, memory issues, and loss of libido. It affects muscle mass and bone health. Progesterone is neuroprotective against brain ageing. It is made during rapid eye movement (REM) sleep. Testosterone strengthens the adrenals, which allows us to deal with stress better.

The immune system is most active at night, and deep sleep is needed for this. During light sleep, the body is healing its detox pathways, as the lymphatic system is most active during sleep: 60% more than in the daytime. This is why when we are ill, we sleep more, and our lymphatic system works overtime fighting infection. Night shift workers have a higher incidence of cardiovascular disease, diabetes, and obesity, suggesting daytime sleeping may cause metabolic conditions. Similarly, people with chronic auto-immune diseases often have poor sleep. Cytokines are made and produced in sleep, which is why we naturally sleep more in the flu season, autumn, and winter to protect the body from viruses.

In the brain, there is a lymphatic system, the glymphatic system (discovered in 2013[10]), where there is a fluid exchange between the spinal fluid (CSF) and the fluid in the brain (ISF). The glymphatic system is regulated during sleep when the brain pulses (expands and contracts). This pumping mechanism removes waste products, fluid, and soluble proteins from the brain. The rate of waste removal is 60% higher in sleep than in waking. One of the brain's waste products is amyloid beta, which is raised in Alzheimer's (see Thinking). The glymphatic system can be impaired following brain injury, stroke, and brain haemorrhage. It is early days in this research, but it can be seen how important good sleep is for brain health, especially as we grow older.

Poor sleep affects insulin resistance, cardiovascular disease, depression, and mood disorders (it is suggested over 90% of mental health conditions are co-concomitant with sleep disorders).[11] Sleep resets the nervous system. Poor sleep affects immune function and lowers life expectancy. Poor sleep often causes a craving for junk foods, especially sweet sugary snacks that 'give you a boost'. In the hierarchy of the foundations of health, sleep is number 1, followed by diet, exercise, and stress reduction. Sleep affects every single cell in the body.

The circadian rhythm (CR) is how the body naturally brings periods of rest and activity to the body. Our physiology is made for optimal sleep. When we wake up and see the sunlight, this stimulates the production of cortisol. CR regulates our sleep patterns. We have a 24-hour internal clock which is controlled by daylight and eating habits. The CR influences our lifespan. Our genes are under circadian control. Light exposure hits the retina, which is transmitted to the superchiasmatic nucleus area of the brain where serotonin is produced into melatonin, which makes you sleepy from the pineal gland is found. Conversely, cortisol wakes us up.

Circadian rhythm allows humans and animals to make the best use of their environment and also regulate internal processes. They are endogenous (controlled from within us) and respond to external stimuli, especially light and temperature. Light exposure is more important to CR than melatonin levels. When the eye sees sunlight, the pineal gland stops producing melatonin (the sleep hormone) and hormones which keep the body awake are produced.

The science of sleep

The suprachiasmatic nucleus (SCN), a brain area directly above the optic chiasm, is presently considered the most important site for melatonin regulation; however, secondary clock systems have been found throughout the body. Cortisol levels rise during the night, peak in the early morning, and slowly run down during the day, circadian prolactin starts being secreted in the afternoon and peaks in the middle of the night, and CR influences the growth hormone at night. Sleepiness increases during the night. REM sleep occurs more during body temperature, minimum within the circadian cycle. Exposure to even small amounts of light during the night can suppress melatonin secretion and increase body temperature and wakefulness. A person in synch with the sun will (during most of the year) fall asleep a few hours after sunset, experience a body temperature minimum at 6 am, and wake up a few hours after sunrise.

Naps

There are different opinions on this, but the consensus is that a short nap, 10–20 minutes, is the optimal time; any longer and the person enters slow-wave sleep, the deepest period of sleep, entering this cycle can make it difficult to wake up and also leave you feeling tired. The siesta habit has been associated with lower rates of coronary artery disease, perhaps due to stress reduction.[12]

Stages of sleep

When you sleep, your brain goes through four cycles in two phases: non-REM sleep and REM sleep. Non-REM sleep happens first and includes three stages; the last two phases of non-rem sleep are when you sleep deeply. REM sleep happens 1–1.5 hours after falling asleep. This is when you have vivid dreams, hence the rapid eye movements. As you sleep, your body cycles through REM and non-REM sleep. A full sleep cycle is around 90 minutes. The first REM cycle is short, but as you sleep deeper the REM cycles grow longer, and you have more REM and less deep sleep.

There are three stages of non-REM sleep.

Stage 1 lasts 5–10 minutes and is 3% of sleep. Here, your body begins to slow down; if you wake up in this phase, you may feel you haven't been asleep at all, and sudden muscle movements may jerk you awake.

Stage 2 is when the recuperation happens. Brain waves become slower, eye movement stops, heart rate falls, and your body temperature decreases, as your body prepares to enter deep sleep.

Stage 3 is deep sleep. The brain produces very slow brain waves, Delta waves. There is no muscle movement or eye movement. It is hard to wake up from this phase, and if you do wake you feel groggy and disorientated. This is where the body repairs and regenerates tissue, builds bone and muscle, and strengthens the immune system.

What the body does when we sleep

Sleep may facilitate the synthesis of molecules that help repair and protect the brain from metabolic end-products generated during waking. Anabolic hormones, such as growth hormones, are secreted more during sleep. The brain concentration of glycogen increases during sleep, and is depleted through metabolism during wakefulness.[13] In this phase, the brain filters out unnecessary information collected during the day. As we age, we get less non-REM, and so sleep less deeply.

In REM sleep, there is increased brain activity and muscle relaxation; there is faster breathing, increased heart rate and blood pressure, and rapid eye movements. Factors which reduce REM sleep are alcohol, tobacco, caffeine, anti-depressants, and temperature (too hot or too cold). In REM sleep, there is memory consolidation memories are moved from short-term storage to long-term. This files away experiences and is very important for dealing with anxious thoughts as our troubles are backed up into the deep brain. We have a 90-minute cycle of light, deep, and REM sleep throughout the night.

The deepest sleep occurs during the early sleeping hours, especially before midnight; then, between 11 pm and 2 am the body falls into a deep sleep. After that time, sleep is lighter. The longer you stay asleep, the greater the REM cycles. Dream recall occurs in deep REM sleep. If you don't have enough REM sleep, recall drops, and you may not remember your dreams.

The ideal amount of sleep is seven to nine hours, depending on the individual on their physiology. It is quite normal to have periods of light sleep within a sleep cycle with tossing and turning.

So, what can we practically take from all this?

Routine

The body has its own internal clock, which is related to nature's clock. So, aim to sleep in darkness and wake up in the light, in winter as dawn is breaking. We sleep deeper in the hours before midnight. Your good sleep routine starts with how you greet the day (see melatonin above). The ideal sleep time is 10 pm to 6 am. As the day wears on, if you feel sleepy have a 'power nap' of no more than 20 minutes.

In the morning: 30 minutes after waking, go outside, and get that sunlight or daylight into your eyes-looking out of the window doesn't work quite the same. Have a morning walk or sit and stare at the world. This tells your CR it's time to get going and you wake up fully. Light is anti-depressive and affects CR, and shuts down the pineal glands' production of melatonin, which means you are not sleepy all day long. Cortisol levels are highest in the morning, giving a prolonged increase in adrenaline to increase energy and high glucose levels for longer periods of time and insulin resistance. Try to spend 10–15 minutes outside; light is more important than exercise to reset CR and produces the right amount of melatonin and serotonin. Don't look at your phone or a screen or TV for 30 minutes. It is important to reset the CR in the morning so that when evening comes you are tired, and the brain starts to build melatonin for the evenings as darkness triggers the pineal gland to release melatonin. Melatonin makes us sleepy. As we age, our melatonin production drops. Melatonin has a positive, curative effect on the brain (as does sleep); it is believed to protect against certain cancers, as tumours grow faster when melatonin levels are low. It also has an anti-inflammatory action and may enhance cytokine production (see Nourishment).

Meditate. Whatever is going on in your life, start the day with a positive mindset. Meditation calms the brain and body, relaxes our brain, and helps to calm the racing mind and uplift sadness (see Happiness).

Eating. Eat good fats, protein, and some carbohydrates and fibre (see Nourishment). Have your last meal at least three hours before bed, ideally at 6 pm; eating late confuses the body about what time of day it is. Try to eat regularly, as the body will be anticipating food (those internal body clocks again). Eat your heaviest foods at lunch and morning. Take your cup of coffee or tea before midday. Leave 12 hours between your last meal and breakfast to give your digestive system a rest (see Nourishment). Digestion works most efficiently 10–4 pm.

Unregulated blood sugar levels can be associated with poor sleep. Waking at 3 am can indicate low blood sugar, and high glucose levels increase cortisol and adrenaline, which can wake us up. Blood glucose waking is a survival mechanism. When the adrenals release adrenaline, we may wake up hungry or think we need to pee when it is the low blood sugar that has woken us up. A handful of nuts before bed may help this.

Detoxing. In Traditional Chinese Medicine (TCM) the hours of the day are related to various organs: between 1–3 am, the liver is most active (detoxifying), and the gall bladder time is between 11 pm–1 am. So, early morning waking may be related to over-toxicity of the body, and too much fire-yang energy. Environmental toxins, drugs, and alcohol are all removed from the system during these hours as the peripheral clock is influenced by non-light factors. In the Action chapter below, there is a list of environmental toxins to consider, especially if sleep issues are of sudden onset and have no other biological cause. Especially check your mattress, as they can give off fumes, so try to get an organic one or a futon. The same applies to sheets and pillows and all bedding, and these can all put a toxic load on your liver.

Exercise

Take exercise, outside if possible, and walking is so good for this. Exercise uses up energy, and it decreases body temperature via sweat. It increases the sleep drive and decreases anxiety levels. Ask yourself, are you fit enough to sleep? With any exercise, consistency is important, and it takes a while to build up your reserves. However, too much exercise can be detrimental. Two hours of high-intensity exercise, especially near bedtime, can cause a decrease in the quality of sleep and show restlessness and more REM sleep. In the afternoon, take a walk, eat lunch outside, or walk for 20 minutes outside to get some more daylight (see Move).

Daylight

Watching the sunrise and sunset over a period of days will reset your CR to fit into the natural rhythm of sleep and wakefulness. Spend time in nature; holidays are great for this. Go camping to connect back to your natural sleep cycle. In the summer, spend 15 minutes out in the sunlight without sunglasses. Vitamin D is made by the body in the presence of sunlight. Vitamin D deficiency is implicated in many diseases and is associated with poor-quality sleep.

Darkness

Change your sleep environment: remove fluorescent lightbulbs and very blue incandescent light bulbs. Put on an orange light in the evening to resemble the setting sun. Put your phone to bed; in the evening, turn off all devices which produce blue light at least two hours before sleep. Blue light stimulates dopamine release, and cortisol which is stimulating. Blue light glasses worn 1–2 hours before bed can help the production of melatonin to encourage sleepiness.

Temperature

Have a bath or shower before bed; this cools your body down which aids sleep. Take a warm shower or cold or a warm bath before sleep; this will lower your body temperature by half a degree, and good sleep is more likely to happen. Body temperature drops significantly during sleep; we are meant to feel slightly cool then. Our core temperature drops at the beginning of sleep and rises around 4 am as we begin to sleep less deeply, ready for a 6 am wake up. When our body cools, it is a sign that the body releases hormones for sleep. The ideal temperature for sleep is 18–20C or 65–72F. Overheating bedrooms can be a cause of sleeplessness.

Emotional causes

Relaxation

Do some deep breathing exercises (see Action). Use breathwork to slow your system down and connect with your deeper self, and slow down a racing mind. Yin yoga may be helpful for chilling out or having an evening walk after 8 pm. Practice active relaxation; we don't need to be busy all the time. Burnout is when we have neglected 'being' by 'doing' too much. Cultivate the gentle and the slow, which nourishes the deeper parts of ourselves. Activities such as being in nature, and comforting activities like reading and drawing or gardening will relax you. Aim to be nourishing yourself all the time.

Control might be an issue for sleeplessness. What does it mean? Is there something you can't fix? Sometimes we compensate during the daytime by being busy, but at night concerns cannot be suppressed, and they bubble up, causing you to wake. For this reason, it is important not to suppress these emotions because as you sleep those emotions and thoughts will disturb your rest. If you have things on your mind, writing in a journal can let all the feelings out before you sleep or if you wake up. Writing down the experiences of the day, a 'brain dump' releases worries and negative thoughts. Practice being positive and focus on something good that happened during the day, however small. In bed, run through the day with gratitude, because there is always something to be grateful for. Or list acts of kindness you have done and received that day (see Happiness).

Information detox

This is important if you have troubled sleep. Limit the time you spend on social media and bad news reports; instead, focus on uplifting content, books, music, and activities which make you feel good. To manage stress, try to do something you love every day, especially before bed, as this lowers cortisol which will stop you from falling asleep and also cause you to wake up multiple times during the night.

Waking up

Sometimes we wake up during the night as it is a quiet time when we can think uninterrupted or even work for a couple of hours. When my daughter was a baby, I went to sleep with her and trained myself to wake up at 3 am to do a couple of hours of work, or simply sit still in silence, before returning to bed to sleep another couple of hours until she woke up. If you can't sleep or you wake up during the night, after 20 minutes or so lying in bed get up and read a dull book or do a puzzle or do something relaxing and then go back to bed when you feel sleepy. If you wake early, it may be your cycle needs adapting. Try an earlier bedtime: 8 pm to 3 am is still seven hours of sleep, and there is something magically peaceful about the earliest hours if you are rested.

Tape your mouth. Putting tape over your mouth, so you breathe through your nose when you sleep activates the parasympathetic nervous system and brings a deep relaxation. (see appendix of suppliers). Obstructive sleep apnoea occurs when the air supply to the lungs is poor, and the lack of oxygen causes us to wake up. This is aggravated by hay fever, colds, allergies, pollen sinuses, enlarged tonsils, chronic infection, and eating lots of dairy, sugar, and alcohol. Sleep apnoea occurs as we age because the muscles in the airways weaken; as we lose muscle tone, our jaw becomes slack and partially blocks the airways. In sleep, we should ideally breathe through the nose; when we breathe through the mouth, it stimulates the sympathetic nervous system's fight-or-flight mechanism.

Mouth breathing is a primary cause of snoring, which can cause disruptions in your sleep and keep you from being fully rested by increasing REM sleep. Nasal breathing while sleeping creates nitrous oxide, which increases blood flow, lowers blood pressure, and improves brain function. Using mouth tape promotes breathing through your nose by gently and comfortably keeping your mouth closed while you sleep.

Herbal helpers

A herbal prescription includes remedies for sleep itself, remedies to tone and soothe the nervous system, remedies to help detoxify of the liver (see Materia Media for details).

For sleep

If insomnia is an occasional problem, then taking a herbal remedy before bed can help to calm the mind and relax the body.

- Lavender essential oil: 10 drops in a warm bath or on the pillow or one drop each on the temples may be enough to relax the mind before sleep.
- Chamomile is gently relaxing and can be taken as a tea and coffee substitute during the afternoon as it calms the body.
- Hops: 5 ml of the tincture taken 30 minutes before bedtime gives a deep relaxation and as a bitter supports the liver in its detoxifying work during the night.

• Linden blossom is a great relaxant, stronger than chamomile, which can be taken throughout the day for anxiety and in the evening as bedtime approaches.

Longer-term treatment (take professional advice)

It may be your adrenals are overstimulated and exhausted. Borage can help with that.

If your nervous system is depleted, then oat straw is a lovely remedy to nourish and build up nerve tissue over a period of time.

Skullcap is especially useful for people who cannot sleep or wake up early because their minds are over-active.

Valerian is found in many over-the-counter herbal sleep remedies. It works really well for most people, but for some people it has the opposite effect, so I tend not to use it.

Passiflora is also a useful remedy for sleep found in many over-the-counter remedies.

Good sleep is our birth-right. We do not have to suffer poor sleep as we age.

CHAPTER 3

Stretch

I may have lost some of you already. If exercise reminds you of freezing on pitches in school sports, I promise you, this is not what I mean. Exercise needs to be enjoyable; otherwise, we won't do it. The secret is to find a type of exercise which you like. There will be one, I promise!

First, the science of what happens in your body when you move it.

Physical exercise modulates the immune system; during and after exercise, pro and anti-cytokines are released, and lymphocytes circulate in the bloodstream in greater numbers making the body more resistant to viruses with moderate, regular exercise.[14]

Exercise has been shown to increase glucose sensitivity and glucose uptake (see Nourishment). Resistance training increases muscle mass, further increasing glucose uptake; this effect can last several hours after exercise. High-intensity Interval Training (HIT), short bursts of exercise, decreases fasting insulin levels. Insulin is associated with metabolic abnormalities, including type 2 diabetes, hypertension, and obesity. Exercise has been shown to reverse insulin sensitivity and the subsequent development of type 2 diabetes. Doing 2.5 hours of exercise a week has been shown to stop this progression; increase this to 4–7 hours to treat obesity.[15]

Resistance training (RT) has a dramatic effect on insulin sensitivity and glucose uptake and is seen to be more effective than aerobic training (AT). Skeletal muscle accounts for 75–95% of glucose uptake; increasing muscle mass can dramatically stabilise blood glucose levels. Combining RT and AT more than doubles the effectiveness of the exercise. Exercise reduces levels of the stress hormone cortisol. Cortisol makes us crave sugars and makes us insulin resistant, and increases belly fat. Exercise has a positive effect on the brain; it reduces depression and anxiety and increases memory strength.

Exercise improves the circulation and the heart and reduces inflammation, which is a cause of high blood pressure and stroke. Exercise balances hormones and so reduces the risk of breast and other common cancers. When you sweat, you release toxins via your skin (the largest organ in your body). Exercise stimulates the function of your colon (evacuation), and regular bowel movements are vital for health. Gentle exercise stimulates the lymphatic system to remove toxins and fluid from the body. Exercise also improves sexual function.

Exercise has a positive effect on the brain as it stimulates the production of brain-derived neurotrophic factor BDMF.[16] BDMF is increased in aerobic training, and it is believed this is why brain health is improved with regular exercise. Short-term exercise improves cognitive function (how well you think, reason, and remember). Long-term exercise improves the plasticity of the brain, and cognitive function and helps to prevent neurological disease. Studies have found[17] that exercise removes the effects of obesity on brain inflammation. Or, to put it another way, lack of exercise and obesity decrease blood flow to the brain, which is one of the causes of Alzheimer's. A study of older people, 60 years+ (51% women) found that increased BMI (body mass index) is associated with decreased CBF_{GM} (grey matter cerebral blood flow), and happily, this was reversible. If the obese people exercised, there was no decrease in CBF_{GM}. Exercise mitigates against weight gain … eat cake and dance!

How is exercise classified? This is one way of measuring the amount of exercise taken by the MET (Metabolic Equivalent Task).[18] High activity is a high-intensity activity for three days per week of 1,500 MET minutes, which can be calculated here.[19] High activity can also be a combination of hard physical activity plus moderate activity and walking every day, or 3,000 MET minutes per week. While moderate levels of activity include 20 minutes of vigorous activity three times a week for 20 minutes duration or moderate activity for 30 minutes every day. A combination of moderate and High Activity exercise accumulates 600 MET minutes per week.

Remember, exercise does not have to be sweaty gyms. Gardening, dancing, swimming, walking, climbing hills, and vigorous house cleaning, can all be included in exercise. Aerobic training may be walking up hills, vigorous housework, cycling, dancing, swimming, and racquet sports. Resistance training is the heavy lifting of the main muscle groups, so gardening, dynamic yoga, weight training, running, rowing, etc. Go outside. We are children of nature, but more and more of us live our lives inside.

Balance

Balance tends to decrease as we grow older, and as we feel less sure on our feet, we do less physical movement, and our balance gets worse. Balance is incredibly important, and poor balance causes falls which are a major cause of mortality in the elderly. Balance is also indicated in a whole variety of other illnesses. The *British Journal of Sports Medicine* did a study[20] which showed the ability to stand on one leg (OLS) for 10 seconds was a predictor of survival in middle-aged and older people. The study looked at 1,702 men and women aged 51–75 (68% male) and found 20.4% were unable to do this. Follow-up after seven years showed 7.2% of those who couldn't do this died compared to 4.6% of those who could.

Balance can be regained with practice. Tai Chi is an excellent exercise for this as there is a lot of bent knee balancing and movement. A study[21] found that doing Tai Chi twice a week increased balance and confidence in older people. Fear of falling and consequent clumsiness is a major health risk in the elderly, Tai Chi involves slow, dance-like movements that strengthen leg muscles, agility, balance, endurance, flexibility, and coordination. The yang style, a simplified form, consists of 24 exercises, developed by the Chinese government. Tai Chi is practised as a public exercise with thousands of people taking part; in the early morning in China, parks and squares are full of Tai Chi devotees. In the study, practising outdoors in a group showed more improvement than solo practice. We are social creatures, go out, meet people, and exercise.

Everyday balance exercises like standing on one leg while you brush your teeth can also help. Also, think about your shoes. A useful book is *Falling Is Not an Option: A Way to Lifelong Balance* by George Locker (see Action). He developed a series of exercises based on Tai Chi for everyone, including people on walkers, to rebuild their balance. Other things that are helpful for improving balance include, is walking on grass, and doing yoga or aerobic dance.

Effect of a sedentary lifestyle

People who do little exercise carry as much health risk as people who eat badly and smoke. Lack of exercise increases the risk of heart disease, cancer, and diabetes. The less exercise you do, the higher the risk of your death.

Practice

Do a seven-minute workout, have a partner, take a 30-minute walk daily, and do fun activities such as dancing, wild swimming, sea bathing, and rambling.

- Make it easy; exercise in a regular class or with a friend.
- Have your kit already laid out.
- Exercise first thing in the morning, as we tend to lose motivation later on in the day.
- Make it enjoyable; dance like nobody is watching.

Walking

The benefits of walking are tremendous, but there is no evidence that we need to walk 10,000 steps; this number was dreamed up as part of an advertising campaign in the 1960s Japan.[22] Recent research has shown a far lower number will give health benefits.[23] The mortality risk was markedly reduced up to about 7,500 daily steps.[24] First, researchers found no minimum threshold for the beneficial effect of step counts on mortality, so any number of steps is better than none. The studies differentiate between ambling to the shops and a purposeful walk in nature, although it may be the case that the major benefit is being in nature, rather than walking.[25] In a study, patients in the hospital were found to recover better and take less pain relief when they had a window facing out on to some trees, than those who had a view of a brick wall. Looking at trees makes you feel and be better.

Nature

Being in nature and absorbing all the atmospheres, sounds, smells, and touch that nature evokes in you has a beneficial effect on health. Exercising while being in nature (green exercise) increases the beneficial effects of exercise.[26] There was a clear effect of both exercise and different scenes on blood pressure, self-esteem, and mood. Exercise alone significantly reduced blood pressure, increased self-esteem, and had a significant positive effect on four of six mood measures. Both rural and urban pleasant scenes produced a significantly greater positive effect on self-esteem than the exercise-only control. The combined positive effect of green exercise on both pleasant rural and urban environments. By contrast, both rural and urban unpleasant scenes reduced the positive effects of exercise on self-esteem. The unpleasant rural scenes had the most dramatic effect, depressing the beneficial effects of exercise on three different measures of mood. It appears that threats to the countryside depicted in unpleasant rural scenes have a greater negative effect on mood than already unpleasant urban scenes. Thus, combining exercise and nature has a beneficial effect on health and mood.

Forest bathing

The Japanese government did research which found that two hours spent forest bathing (being in beautiful nature) it has nothing to do with swimming, reduced blood pressure, lowered cortisol levels, and improved concentration and memory. Chemicals released by trees called phytoncides have anti-microbial properties and so help support the immune system. Consequently, the Japanese government incorporated *shinrin-yoku* (forest bathing) into their national health system. Forest bathing is not a hike; it's not exercise; it's not a nature walk; it is like a mindfulness meditation, an exercise to wake up the senses by being in the present moment and closing the eyes and hearing, smelling and sense the trees and nature all around you. You may add a gentle guided meditation to still the mind and be present. Then walk very slowly along the forest, noticing everything, leaves stirring, the breeze, sounds of birds and insects, communing with the trees and hugging them. Immerse yourself in the sensory experience and allow nature to still the mind and heal the body.

Social prescribing

In the bio-psycho-social model of health, a holistic practice offers solutions which are extra-medical,[27] for example, green exercise and forest bathing. It is estimated that around 20% of patients consult their general practitioner (GP) for what is primarily a social problem (Low Commission, 2015). Referral to a social prescribing service could reduce this pressure. Following referral, there was a 28% reduction in GP visits and an average of 24% reduction in A&E visits. Although more research is needed, taking a holistic view of health makes sense. Exercise in nature, or at least looking at nature is part of the mix.

Parkrun[28]

Parkruns are free, weekly, community events all around the world. Saturday morning events are 5k runs and take place in parks and open spaces. On Sunday mornings, there are 2k junior parkruns for children aged 4 to 14. Parkrun is designed for non-athletes; there is no time limit to finish the run, no competition, and no one finishes last. Parkruns are open to everyone, and offer a form of exercise which is inclusive: you can jog, walk, run, volunteer as a steward, or watch the races. There are over a thousand parkruns happening around the country. Group exercise like parkruns encourages people at all levels of fitness to learn new ways to exercise, enjoy being in nature (they happen in parks) and socialise. Parkrun is free. They have a YouTube channel where participants speak about their experiences.[29]

Dancing

There is a saying among Native Americans, when a person falls ill, the healer asks, 'When did you stop dancing?' Dancing is something[30] that requires several complex skills, including spatial awareness (not treading on your partner's toes), movement timing and execution (auditory and motor integration), memory (to remember the steps), and listening (to the music). Dancing, then, increases coordination, and the strengthens the part of the brain concerned with planning and movement. Dancing affects the hippocampus of the brain. We lose 2 or 3% of the hippocampus each decade as we age; over 70 years we can lose 1% per year. This loss is particularly rapid in dementia and Alzheimer's. The hippocampus grows in response to certain physical activities which have mental challenges (dance, yoga, Tai Chi, etc.). Studies on healthy adults over 63 years who did aerobics classes twice a week showed increased hippocampus volume; the effect may be linked to improved balance.[31] Dancing is great exercise, and it improves wellbeing, happiness, and creativity.[32]

Degeneration of white matter (WM) in the brain is associated with dementia and cognitive decline in older people. A study on exercise in older adults found that dancing which combined aerobic exercise and cognitive functions, reduced WM decline more than other forms of exercise like walking, cycling, and aerobics. Researchers have found ballroom dancing reduces cognitive decline, and dance classes in residential homes reduces depression. Dance increases the circulation to the brain, which affects the speed at which we process information. Particularly effective in preventing cognitive decline were group dances, like folk dances, where people wove in and out, and there was no leader.[33] (See the chapter on Fun for more).

Exercise, then, is one of the three pillars of health.

CHAPTER 4

Thinking

> The brain is like a 100 billion electric jellyfish crammed into a skull that's floating in clear liquid, spraying chemicals and electricity like it's an aurora borealis. If we knew we are like that in our skulls, we might see our minds and behaviour differently … there are brain cells which are dormant until you have a certain stress, and that's the cue for them to activate. If the stress is too high, they stay dormant. If there isn't any stress, they stay dormant. So, if we start to think of our brains as gardens, it fits more with the patterns of life.
>
> Rahul Jandial, MD, PhD, Neurosurgeon.[34]

People worry about the degeneration of the brain as they age, but as the quote above shows our brains are like gardens; if they are full of weeds, the good plants choke and do not thrive. Gardens require sunlight, water, and nutrients. As I hope I showed in the previous chapters, what we eat and how we rest and move all have a profound effect on the health of our body, and our brains are no exception.

We learnt about the gut microbiome and how insulin resistance, especially, has an effect on inflammation. Twenty-five per cent of the glucose in the body is found in the brain; it is a glucose-rich site. What loves glucose? Unhealthy bacteria.

The 'gut-brain' is really one thing, because your brain talks to your gut and your gut talks to your brain. The gut-brain, or the second brain, is a nervous system with as many neurotransmitters or more than your brain. There is a conversation that happens between your gut and brain. When your gut's unhappy and inflamed, your brain's going to be unhappy and inflamed. The gut-brain and brain connection optimises digestion and may remove the SIBO (Small Intestine Bacterial Overgrowth), which causes digestive disturbances and conditions such as irritable bowel syndrome.

We think diseases of the brain are mental issues, arising from feelings and emotions, but actually most causes of brain disease are biological. We know thoughts and feelings can affect biology, but now, due to work on the microbiome, we know your biology can affect your thoughts and feelings.

Every second there are 37 billion-billion chemical reactions happening in your body; they all require nutrients for co-factors to run everything. One-third of your DNA codes for enzymes, and enzymes are catalysts which run these chemical reactions. Every enzyme needs co-enzymes to function, and co-enzymes require vitamins and minerals to work optimally.

What does your brain need? First, it needs a good diet, exercise, restful sleep, stress reduction, and relaxation. Then there are supplements which enhance brain activity, multivitamins, Omega 3 fats (1 g daily), magnesium, Vitamin D, and methylated nutrients, which we discuss below.

Your brain is made up of mostly Omega 3 fats; 60% of your brain is DHA.[35] Clearly, a brain low in Omega 3 fats will be operating at a sub-par level. Low Omega 3 levels are found in the brains of people suffering from Alzheimer's, Parkinson's disease, depression, and bipolar disease. Eating more Omega 3 fats, in food and supplements, has been found to improve these conditions. Omega 3 fats support brain function, mood, and regulate the metabolism, cool off inflammation and help in diabetes and cardiovascular disease. Originally, we got Omega 3 fats from wild fatty fish, from wild animals, and wild plants (see Action for foods high in Omega 3). Ideally, eat 1–2 g of Omega 3 fat per day.

Omega 6 is found in cheap oils like sunflower and soya oil and in most processed foods, and in animal food (especially in the meat and dairy industries). Omega 6 produces prostaglandins in the body, which can be pro-inflammatory and increase the production of endocannabinoids, which are also pro-inflammatory. Omega 3 produces chemicals which block these inflammatory responses.

Saturated fat

Coconut oil, MCT (Medium Chain Triglyceride) oil,[36] and eggs stimulate the body's production of ketones. A ketogenic diet reduces inflammation and increases energy production. This helps reduce the production of free radicals and stimulates brain cell repair. It has been suggested that MCT oil improves cognitive function in dementia patients. For these saturated fats to do their good work, they should not be eaten with a diet high in sugar and simple carbohydrates (HPFs) or processed, cheap meat, because these have an inflammatory effect which counteracts the benefit of the saturated fats.

Magnesium

Magnesium is a mineral which is vital for overall health. It is a co-factor in over 300 enzyme systems, which regulate protein synthesis, control of blood glucose, regulation of blood pressure, and energy production in the body. Magnesium helps the development of bone tissue and muscle and nerve function, as well as the synthesis of DNA and RNA, the antioxidant glutathione, and the transport of calcium and potassium across cell membranes which support the nervous system, muscle contraction, and normal heart rhythm. Magnesium calms the brain down and promotes restful sleep. The suggested amounts range between 4–6 mg daily.

Vitamin D

Vitamin D is vital for brain health; like magnesium, it is involved in hundreds of gene expression enzymes, and it regulates the function of your immune system and also cognitive function. Vitamin D is made on the skin in the presence of sunlight. It has long been known that Vitamin D is important for bone health, but low levels of this hormone-like vitamin have been found in cardiovascular disease, cancer, stroke, and metabolic disorders, including diabetes.[37] Cognitive impairment, dementia, psychosis, and autism have been added to the list of symptoms of low Vitamin D levels.[38] Vitamin D receptors are widespread in brain tissue, and Vitamin D in its biologically active form (1,25(OH) (2) D3) has shown neuroprotective effects, including the clearance of amyloid plaques, a hallmark of Alzheimer's disease.[39] Recent studies have confirmed an association between cognitive impairment, dementia, and Vitamin D deficiency. Vitamin D was reported to modulate the biosynthesis of neurotransmitters and neurotrophic factors; moreover, its receptor was found in the central nervous system.[40] The daily dose of Vitamin D is 400 units. However, because Vitamin D is fat-soluble, it is stored in the body, and overdosing is possible. Follow the dose guidelines or consult an expert. Foods high in Vitamin D include salmon, egg yolk, shellfish, and mushrooms (see Action).

Methylation

Methylation is a constantly changing process in our cells which responds to dietary and environmental factors (epigenetics) and affects gene expression in the body.

What is methylation?[41]

In methylation, a carbon methyl group is transferred from one molecule to another. This either activates the molecule or deactivates it. Several enzymes[42] facilitate methylation. Nutrients such as B12, B6, magnesium, sulphur and zinc, choline, betaine, methionine, and folate support methylation.[43]

Methylation is needed for cell division, detoxification, and hormone biotransformation, neurotransmitter growth, histamine clearance, central nervous system development, myelination of peripheral nerves, DNA and RNA synthesis, and phospholipid synthesis.

One of the best biomarkers (indicators in the body/cells) for ageing is changes in DNA methylation. DNA methylation and epigenetic alterations have been directly linked to longevity in a wide array of organisms, ranging in complexity from yeast to humans.[44]

Because there has been some research that folate supplements can cause hypermethylation, it is recommended that a healthy diet is the best way to support methylation, with the added benefit that a good diet also provides phytonutrients, vitamins, and minerals, which also support methylation. Pesticides can affect methylation, so eat organic whenever you can (see Action for dirty dozen and clean 15). Certain foods increase the action of DNMT (DNA methyltransferase[45]) enzymes which carry out methylation. These include curcumin, ellagic acid, lycopene, quercetin, resveratrol, rosmarinic acid, and sulforaphane.

Foods supporting methylation[46]

Dark leafy greens like broccoli, kale, and spinach contain high levels of folate.

Cruciferous vegetables are methylation adaptogens (they contain folate and sulforaphane). These include broccoli, cabbage, Brussels sprouts, kale, cauliflower, and rocket. Beetroot (including the green tops) contains high levels of betaine, a choline metabolite which acts as a methyl donor.

Lentils and pinto beans and peas contain high levels of folate and molybdenum, copper and B1.

Okra is high in B6, B1, copper, magnesium, and manganese which support methylation.

Mushrooms, especially shiitake mushrooms, may be methylation adaptogens as they reduce homocysteine (an unhelpful compound which may cause heart disease and deplete levels of B6, B12, and folate). They also contain B5, niacin, riboflavin, B6, B12, copper, and selenium.

Seeds like pumpkin are high in folate, magnesium, and choline; sunflower seeds are high in B1, B6, magnesium, copper, folate, selenium, and betaine, while sesame seeds are high in choline, thiamine, manganese, magnesium, zinc, copper, niacin, and folate.

Turmeric has high levels of curcumin and choline, which are methylation adaptogens.

Rosemary (both fresh and dried) contains rosmarinic acid, another methylation adaptogen that regulates the enzyme DNMT.

Berries such as blackberries, goji berries, black currents, blueberries, strawberries, and raspberries contain many helpful phytonutrients and anthocyanins, chlorogenic acid, ellagic acid, and quercetin. They are epigenetically active, making them potent methylation adaptogens.

Green tea contains epigallocatechin gallate, catechins, and other flavanols that may also benefit methylation activity. Researchers suspect that these phytonutrients may be able to favourably impact tumour suppressor genes via methylation.

Coffee also contains chlorogenic acid[47] (see Fun for details).

Animal liver is a methylation promoter, but it needs to be organic as any chemicals given to the animal (often dairy cattle are given anti-biotics) are processed in the liver and may leave a residue there.

Genes

Methylation constitutes the best-studied, and likely most resilient of many mechanisms controlling gene expression.[48] Methylation is a constantly changing process in our cells which responds to dietary and environmental factors (epigenetics) and affects gene expression in the body.

In methylation, a carbon methyl group is transferred from one molecule to another. This either activates the molecule or deactivates it. Several enzymes[49] facilitate methylation. Nutrients such as B12, B6, magnesium, sulphur and zinc, choline, betaine, methionine, and folate support methylation.[50]

Methylation is needed for cell division, detoxification and hormone biotransformation, neurotransmitter growth, histamine clearance, central nervous system development, myelination of peripheral nerves, DNA and RNA synthesis, and phospholipid synthesis.

One of the best biomarkers (indicators in the body/cells) for ageing is changes in DNA methylation. DNA methylation and epigenetic alterations have been directly linked to longevity in a wide array of organisms, ranging in complexity from yeast to humans.[51]

Because there has been some research that folate supplements can cause hypermethylation, it is recommended that a healthy diet is the best way to support methylation, with the added benefit that it supplies phytonutrients, vitamins, and minerals, which also support methylation.

Pesticides can affect methylation, so eat organic whenever you can (see Action for dirty dozen and clean 15). Certain foods increase the action of DNMT enzymes which carry out methylation, and they include curcumin, ellagic acid, lycopene, quercetin, resveratrol, rosmarinic acid, and sulforaphane.

A study with mice who were genetically reared to be fat, blonde, and prone to diabetes looked at the effect of diet on their genes. The control group were fed the normal diet, and the

experimental group were fed high methylation foods containing B6, B12, folate, etc. The genetic picture of the experimental
group grew up to become brown, skinny, and healthy mice.
Their diet changed their genes.

A study[52] working with healthy males ages 50–75 over
an eight-week period, found they were able to reduce their
biological age with a diet low in carbohydrates and high
in DMNT-promoting foods, sleep, stress reduction, fasting,
and exercise plus probiotics and phytonutrient supplements.
They tested the genome-wide methylation from saliva (Horvath
DNAmAge clock (2013)) and found a 3.23 decrease in
DNAmAge compared with the controls. The DNAmAge clock
shows that 60% of CpG sites lose methylation with age which
promotes inflammation through increased cytokines, while there
was a 40% increase in methylation in areas concerned with tumour
suppression genes (which suppresses their activity). This has
led some researchers to propose that ageing itself has its basis
in epigenetic changes (including methylation changes) over time.

Methylation nutrients are also important for brain function,
and they include Vitamin B12, folate, and B6. These all regulate neurotransmitters, how nerve cells communicate with
each other, cognitive (thinking) function, dealing with oxida-
tive stress, and building glutathione levels.

Glutathione

Glutathione is an antioxidant found in animals, plants, and
fungi; it helps to prevent damage to the cells caused by free
radicals and heavy metals. Levels of glutathione are reduced
by stress, poor diet, and environmental toxins, and levels
reduce with age, making the elderly more susceptible to cell

damage. Glutathione is produced in the body, especially the liver, and is made from three amino acids, glutamine, glycine, and cysteine. Glycine and cysteine supplements improve insulin resistance, fat burning, and peripheral circulation. They also stimulate immunity and protect cell mitochondria.

Herbs which support glutathione include milk thistle and turmeric (see Materia Medica).

The mitochondria are the energy cells of the body; low brain energy, brain fog, Alzheimer's, Parkinson's and depression are associated with underperforming mitochondria. Mitochondria nutrients such as CoQ10, GABA theanine from green tea, and the herb rhodiola all increase mitochondria activity. As we age, our mitochondria weaken.

Homocystine is an amino acid and is broken down in the body by vitamins B6, B12, and folate. High levels of homocysteine have been associated with an increased risk of dementia, heart disease, depression, and stroke.

The microbiome: gut-brain links[53]

The word microbiome comes from the Greek (micros-small) (bios-life). A microbiome is a collection of small organisms that live together. We have a microbiome in the gut which scientists have discovered communicates with the brain, and furthermore disturbances in the gut microbiome have been seen to worsen the severity of many neurological disorders, including neurodegenerative diseases. It has been widely observed that there were distinct microbiome profiles and dysbiosis (a disequilibrium in the gut flora) seen in patients suffering from Alzheimer's disease, Parkinson's disease, amyotrophic lateral sclerosis, and multiple sclerosis. Why this should be is unclear.

Treatments aimed at re-establishing the gut microbiome, such as antibiotic therapy, faecal microbiota transplants, and psycho-biotics, have had limited effects. The gut microbiome of Alzheimer's disease (AD) patients showed a decrease in the diversity of the gut microbes compared with healthy controls. It is possible that the amyloid plaques found in AD come from pathogenic microbes from the gut.[54]

These gut microbes are vital for human health, energy production, biosynthesis of vitamins, protection against pathogens, and immunity. Alterations of this complex ecosystem are associated with inflammatory bowel disease (IBD), insulin resistance, obesity, and metabolic diseases like diabetes.

I suggest that diet then, and consequent gut health, is crucial to brain health.

Connection

Our brain connects us to our environment and other people. What we eat controls how we think and our behaviour choices. Highly processed food (HPF) is addictive; we literally rewire our brains to crave bad food. Overeating and bingeing make connections to the fear-based and reactive (habit pattern) parts of the brain which also control selfish and narcissistic behaviour. So, eating when we are sad, for comfort and when we are angry calms us down. Pathways develop in our brains which then become habits; we do them without thinking. Ask any ex-smoker about breaking habitual patterns they have developed with cigarettes. Like smoking after meals, when making phone calls, after a row, etc., and they will tell you how often they don't even remember picking the cigarette up; it is an unconscious habit. With these habits, we get a dopamine reward (the feel-good chemical), so and the next time we finish a meal, or make a call, we unconsciously reach for a cigarette. This is how we rewire our brains because the brain and its neurons are plastic or changeable. This is good news as far as using the brain is concerned, because if we can rewire it for harmful habits, we can rewire it to make good choices.

After a stroke, which is a catastrophic event in the brain, patients can learn to walk, think, and speak again, which demonstrates how we can grow new neural pathways in our brains. These neural pathways are habitual actions we take, which become automatic, like walking, holding a cup, or using a knife and fork. We can re-programme our brains to do healthy things, sleep, exercise, and good diet, which is just as easy to slip into as bad habits. It has recently been discovered, that after a stroke we repair and rebuild brain tissue; it was previously believed that once destroyed the brain could not repair itself. So even if we have noticed cognitive decline, we can reverse it.[55]

Rewiring your brain

The brain loves repetition; remember how small children learn: they endlessly repeat the same processes until they have mastered them. Learning is the same for adults. We may have been lucky to have a good memory as adults, but as we age memory needs to be worked at. We have talked about the physical body, diet, supplements, etc., and this section looks at the brain as a muscle which we can train and invigorate.

Use it or lose it.

As adults, we fall into routines, doing similar things every day; we often operate on automatic. In these conditions, the brain rests. The brain is a super-efficient organ, and it doesn't waste energy unnecessarily. If thinking and actions become automatic, a large part of the brain goes to sleep. After many years, those sleeping parts of the brain turn off entirely.

Our brains are designed to be used right up until we die. They can function well, even after their physical health declines. However, if a routine life is sending large parts of our brains to sleep, the body can outlive the brain, which is what we see in dementia and Alzheimer's.

So, what to do? Learn something, read, and stretch your brain. Food, exercise, and sleep all prime your brain for action. Go to classes like the University of the Third Age, talk to people out of your social group, and take up drawing and painting and other creative work (including gardening), which activates these underused parts of our brain. Music, especially learning to play an instrument, is a wonderful workout for the brain.

Popular science divides the brain into left and right hemi-spheres, but there is constant communication between the two sides. When we become interested in an idea, both sides of the brain are triggered. When we prepare to do a task, it is the left brain that activates, while the right brain takes goes into deep thought to mull over an idea and to get an 'aha' idea of what to do. The left brain checks this solution out. Will it work? Then both the left and right sides of the brain do the work.[56]

Men's sheds, knitting groups, cooking, gardening, sewing, painting, walking, foraging, chess, life drawing, model mak-ing, language learning, the list is endless. If you are at a loss, remember what you loved as a child and find a way to do that now. Your brain will thank you (see Fun).

Amyloid patches and Alzheimer's

The drug company Pfizer invested heavily in Alzheimer's research; imagine the money that could be made if they invented a magic pill to cure it. However, a succession of drugs failed in trials to improve Alzheimer's symptoms. The majority of the trials were aimed at reducing amyloid patches, which are found in the brains of sufferers. The steady drip of failure suggests that drugs aimed at eliminating amyloid plaques, the biological markers of Alzheimer's, are unlikely ever to succeed and that new approaches are needed.[57]

Why is this?

Because there is no magic bullet for the treatment of Alzheimer's and Parkinson's, and no drug that can fix this, instead, a multi-dimensional approach study, such as the Finger Study is recommended,[58] which highlights diet, exercise, stress reduction, social, and cognitive approaches to preventing and improving neurological diseases such as Alzheimer's.

Pfizer has now admitted failure and abandoned clinical trials to find a drug to cure Alzheimer's disease.

More worryingly, clinical trials with Alzheimer's disease patients generally allow participants to continue receiving their usual medication, including cholinesterase inhibitors (ChEls) and memantine, if the dose is stable. After the trials, the patients' brains showed that people on their Alzheimer's medication showed a greater rate of decline on cognitive testing than those not taking these drugs.[59]

Translated: these medicines may actually increase Alzheimer's symptoms (cognitive decline).

Alzheimer's: type 3 diabetes?

Diets high in simple carbohydrates with a reduction in healthy fat and low dietary fibre cause high blood sugar levels, which cause inflammation throughout the body, including the brain. Inflammation, particularly from gluten-containing grains, makes holes in the gut wall, which allows dangerous chemicals to enter the bloodstream and stimulate the immune cells to start an inflammatory response by creating cytokines to neutralise these toxins by increasing the production of free radicals which damage proteins, fat, DNA, and the mitochondria. The healthy gut is diverse, like the ecosystem of a rainforest, the unhealthy gut, is denuded like a monocrop.

A study of insulin resistance examined if there was a correlation with β-amyloid plaques and found levels substantially higher in those with greater insulin resistance. The amyloid has been the focus of the pharmaceutical industry (see above). But amyloid production is not the problem; it is instead a reaction to infections like herpes simplex virus, and chlamydia, organisms which colonise the brain, causing inflammation. Especially interesting is that a correlation has been found between gum and tooth disease (inflammation) and dementia and arthritis, the mechanism is not clear, but it may be the inflammatory substances are passing into the brain from the mouth.[60]

Sleep is hugely involved in reducing inflammation in the brain, enhancing the excretion of harmful substances from the brain, and the glymphatic system, and triaging our day-to-day experiences where they will be meaningful to us (see Rest).

Grain brain

As we said at the beginning of this chapter, the brain contains 25% of the body's glucose. When we become insulin resistant, through a high sugar and refined carbohydrate diet (see Nourishment), the blood-brain barrier, which allows glucose to enter the brain, becomes compromised. The reduced uptake of glucose by the brain is one predictor of Alzheimer's 20–30 years later. Ketones can be used as fuel for brain cells. Good fat is an alternative energy source for the brain; glucose is not the only way that the brain can make energy (as previously believed). The brain can use fats as a super fuel (see this as a biological hunter-gatherer mechanism for emergency fuel supply). Brain scans of Alzheimer's sufferers showed non-active areas, which were not utilising glucose; it was previously believed these neurones were dead. However, when you supply ketones (in the form of MCT oil) to the body, these neurons start working again. The cells were resting as there was an inadequate energy supply.

Food for the brain, indeed.

This chapter gave you the science behind your brain. Things which hurt the brain. Things we can eat to heal the brain. Things we can do to maximise the brain and its functions.

CHAPTER 5

Happiness

The more you do something, the more you do something.

We have three brains; the oldest and original part of the brain is found in the brainstem. This part controls basic functions in the body such as digestion, blood pressure, breathing, heartbeat, and the 'fight-or-flight' mechanism. Reptiles and birds have the same brain (probably traced back to the time of the dinosaurs). This brain works automatically; under normal circumstances, we don't have conscious input into how it operates.

The next part is the limbic system, which is above the brainstem and receives messages from it. It is here our emotions are formed, which respond to sensations automatically and form part of our survival mechanism, such as we see something terrifying, and we feel fear and run away, or feel anger and fight. It signals survival mechanisms such as responses to hunger and pain, and survival emotions, such as anger, pleasure, sexual arousal, and sleepiness. Dopamine is released by this brain, and endorphins which are naturally produced opiates, which give us feelings of pleasure. Dopamine has been called the 'reward system', which governs habits and ensures we receive instant gratification for these survival needs. This is the biological source of addictive behaviours.

The amygdala is part of the limbic system and is concerned with fear responses. When this part of the brain becomes damaged, people become fearless (or reckless) and aggressive. When fearful experiences occur, the amygdala communicates with the nearby hippocampus (the memory centre), so we remember this experience. Then the hippocampus talks to the highest level of the brain, the prefrontal cortex, which assimilates this memory and adds it to previous memories. This process allows us to remember threats and react to them instinctively; for example, someone shouting causes us to move away before the thought to do so has been formed. Panic attacks and OCD (obsessive-compulsive disorder) responses come from this mechanism. Fear responses and aggressive responses come from the amygdala. Poor impulse control, depression, anxiety, and PTSD (post-traumatic stress disorder) are all associated with overstimulation of the amygdala.

The highest part of the brain, on top of the limbic system, is found in mammals, the cerebral cortex. The common image of the folds of the brain is what the cerebral cortex looks like; the more folds there are, the more complex the brain is. The cerebral cortex is the reasoning, thinking brain, where we can plan, make complex decisions, and use abstractions and logic. The cerebral cortex is intended to regulate the limbic system, called top-down brain functioning. The rationality of the cerebral cortex gave us superior survival skills as mammals; we avoid rather than react to harm.

Within the cortex is the prefrontal cortex, which is unique to humans and comprises 10% of the volume of the brain. It is like the conductor of an orchestra which mediates and harmonises the other parts of the brain. The cortex and the amygdala are in constant contact with each other as we deal with sensory input. When the cerebral cortex is dominant, we are rational, compassionate, and empathic; when the amygdala dominates, we are ruled by fight-or-flight emotions, such as anxiety, aggression, and selfishness.[61]

As you would expect, stimulating the prefrontal cortex increases self-regulation and self-control. It is this mechanism which comes into play when someone annoys us. We may feel like punching them (amygdala), but the prefrontal cortex recommends we restrain ourselves and use language or logical thought to express our feelings, instead of acting out the 'primitive' emotions of the amygdala to fight back, which the cortex analyses may cause more danger in the long run. The cortex plans and strategises and the amygdala reacts.

Prolonged stress, such as exposure to violence or abuse, particularly in childhood, overstimulates the amygdala. We grow up in a continual state of stress, in fight-or-flight mode, which makes us reactive, aggressive, and panicked. The prefrontal cortex does not have the opportunity to mediate these powerful emotions, so they become habitual and automatic responses to any perceived threat or stressor.

The plasticity of the brain and its ability to make new neural pathways, means we can re-train our brain to use the prefrontal cortex rather than the amygdala, because the amygdala response is a habit, and habits can be changed. Things that stimulate the prefrontal cortex to override the amygdala include meditation, time in nature, sleep, psychoactive mushrooms, and a good diet.

Psilocybin[62] has been found to increase the nerve connections in the prefrontal cortex with just one dose, and the effects lasted over a month. Clinical trials with the mushroom at UCL are ongoing for chronic depression and have shown great success with patients suffering from chronic, long-term, drug-resistant depression.[63] Psilocybin is illegal in the UK it has recently been licensed for use in Australia. In the Netherlands, Dr Gabor Mate leads a course in using the truffles of Psilocybin,[64] those parts that grow underground, which are legal in that country.

Meditation also affects the prefrontal cortex and the amygdala.[65] Mindfulness Meditation increases the thickness of the prefrontal cortex, and reduces the shrinkage often associated with ageing. Beginning a meditation practice in old age has a pronounced effect on the brain.[66] Heart-focused meditation regulates emotional reactions from the amygdala, so we respond more from our cerebral cortex with reasoned, logical, compassionate responses. Subjects in a US study meditated for 40 minutes per day. Their practice involved non-judgemental awareness of present-moment stimuli without analysis; this markedly improved their brain health (see Action).

Yoga also affects the cerebral cortex.[67] Analysis of brain activity during an Ashtanga Yoga series 1 practice, found increased prefrontal lobe activity (cerebral cortex). Ashtanga, which is a combination of movement (asana), breathwork (pranayama), and focus (drishti), has been found to improve depression, anxiety, stress, and PTSD and decrease glucose metabolism, which is associated with improved regulation of negative emotions. Improved cognitive performance of the elderly probably is believed to be due to increased blood flow to the prefrontal cortex.[68]

Studies as to what harms the brain are just beginning. Dr Perlmutter (*Brainwash* 2020) illustrates how our modern lifestyle privileges the amygdala over the cerebral cortex. This starts with the pleasure centre in the brain. We respond to pleasure by releasing dopamine from the midbrain, and it travels to the amygdala and the hippocampus (emotion and memory) and the *nucleus accumbens* (where we experience pleasure) and from there to the cerebral cortex (decisions). So, we feel pleasure, remember it, and then decide to repeat the process.

Dopamine stimulates craving. Endogenous opioids (made by the body), produce feelings of pleasure (Perlmutter, 2020: 40). The amygdala, hippocampus, prefrontal cortex, and *nucleus accumbens* all have dopamine receptors, so all the pathways to pleasure-seeking, remembering the experience, choosing more of the experience, and feeling soothed, produce a craving for more of the same. This is how addiction is born. The reward pathway, once activated, continues, and the craving becomes habitual and automatic.

The brain is self-regulatory; when it records high levels of dopamine in the blood, it reduces the amount of dopamine secreted in response to the stimulus and the number of receptors for dopamine. So, the next dopamine hit won't be so strong; more of the stimulus is needed to get the same response and a tolerance is built up, and more is needed to have the same effect. It is not only the obvious drugs that have this dopamine effect; any behaviour which gives us pleasure can turn into craving, and then addiction, sugar, junk food, TV, social media, and sex all stimulate the addiction pathway.

When we feel anxious, cortisol is secreted, which starts the 'fight-or-flight' mechanism. Adrenaline increases heart rate and blood flow, and blood glucose is sent to the muscles, so the body can fight or run away to safety. This stress-response pathway is hardwired in our nervous system to ensure our survival. The amygdala activates these responses, and the cerebral cortex withdraws, as we need to think fast and react, rather than deliberate. As a consequence, when we are anxious, we make hasty and irrational decisions.

With chronic stress, we live more from the reactive, irrational amygdala than the cooler, calmer cerebral cortex. This eventually leads to changes in the cortex, so we are less able to suppress the primitive emotions of rage and fear, and we crave pleasure to soothe ourselves. We get stuck in these bad habits in this neural feedback loop, and our anxiety, aggression, and depression become habitual.

What builds stress? Poor sleep, poor diet, social media, and TV. Poor sleep increases cortisol levels which are associated with depression; poor diet increases blood sugar and is initially stimulating, but in the long-term depression by affecting serotonin levels and causes brain inflammation which has been found in people suffering from depression. Inflammation affects our use of the cerebral cortex because the body is in a constant state of stress, and so the amygdala is overstimulated at the expense of the cortex (Perlmutter, p. 46). As we have seen previously, chronic inflammation is found in the brains of Alzheimer's patients and is also found in chronic anxiety and depression. If the amygdala increases and the cortex weakens, our emotions and behaviours change; we become less rational, logical, and calm, and more fearful, hedonistic, and aggressive. Sugar stimulates dopamine, and so it is easily addictive through the reward pathways.

Inflammation affects the brain's response to social media and causes dopamine surges, did people like my post? Has anyone texted me? How many likes do I have? TV, especially the news, is unfailingly negative and affects our mood.[69] News focuses on the personal, and is biased against the community, and favours selfishness and greed. News is digested in bite size, so we can watch for longer than reading books or articles which require thinking (cortex) (see Fun on reading and brain health). Soundbites and clickbait stimulate the amygdala (fear, anger, stress), which releases cortisol bringing the physical effects above. Social media and the news stimulates fear, aggression, tunnel-vision, and desensitisation, and feed our cognitive bias; as we react more and analyse less, and we search out (or are presented with via x), presenting other stories which confirm our beliefs. This leads to groupthink, where we irrationally believe things we would dismiss if we had the time to analyse things properly.

Thinking is a slower process than reacting. Bite-sized news and social media interrupt our thought processes, so we jump to conclusions. It also affects our memory as the pathway between short-term and long-term memory is disrupted when we are constantly interrupted. This disrupted concentration reduces our ability to concentrate and lowers comprehension. The more news we consume, the more the neural pathways of skimming and multitasking are developed (limbic system), and the less we are able to concentrate when we read long passages or are presented with complex arguments.

Clickbait is a dopamine button. News makes us passive as it is mostly about things we cannot influence and presents a world-view which is pessimistic, desensitised, fatalistic, and cynical. And as we have discovered, the more negative you feel, the more negative you become. Investigative journalism requires time and is vital, especially as the new-politics–big-business pipeline funnels most negative news content and filters out the good and wholesome news.

Commonly we reach for high carbohydrates or HPFs (highly processed foods) in snacks, takeaways, alcohol, sugary snacks, and binge-watching TV to 'relax'. We watch on average 144 minutes of live TV in the UK every day; that figure rises to five hours on all audio-visual content.[70] All of these engage the amygdala and inhibit the cerebral cortex, so short-term pleasure is overrides long-term happiness.[71] If you eat processed foods or HPFs, you have an increased risk of depression; food and drink which spikes blood glucose also increase the risk of depression.[72]

Depression and grief

Getting older can be depressing when loved ones die or friends move away. Physical ill health can isolate us, and pain and limited mobility can make us irritable and sad. Retirement and less family responsibility can make us feel redundant and struggle to find a role and meaning in our lives.

Depression is a psycho-social disease. The medical professional has made depression a biological condition which can be 'fixed' with drugs. Sometimes drugs do help when the depression is so severe, and we cannot function. Generally, though, depression is a reaction or symptom of dis-ease in our world.

My favourite book on depression is *Reasons to Stay Alive* by Matt Haig.[73] He wrote this as a young man with acute, debilitating depression. Read his journey if you are interested, but what he discovered is the same that psychologist Dorothy Rowe[74] found out in the 1980s, depression can be fixed with physical and psycho-spiritual approaches. Both Haig and Rowe recommended running, yoga, and meditation, all of which calm the mind and situate the person inside their body, the 'Be Here Now' techniques, which prayer and contemplation across all spiritual disciplines recommend.[75] These help us to be aligned (situated out of our heads into the here and now), in touch with spirit (or whatever your belief system is) and find a reason for living. Rowe suggests depression has its roots in childhood and our desire to be loved and accepted, by 'being good', which in our culture is working to please everyone around us. Rowe argues for psychology and not drug therapy for depression and does not see depression as an illness but a life crisis. The sufferer has lessons to learn about how to live a happy life on their terms. Rowe insists this is achieved not by avoiding emotional pain but by feeling it and at the same time not making rules about what emotional pain means for the future (e.g. I will always be like this, the pain will never end, etc., etc).

Meditation and prayer have similar aims. They focus on the person to be present in their life (rather than dwelling on the past or fearing the future). Their aim is for the person to accept they are good and deserving of love just because they are.

Triggers for depression are often past experiences of loss, abandonment, and rejection which were repressed rather than expressed. This results in these feelings continuing to resonate in our emotions and undermine our self-esteem. As a result, when a new crisis or challenge occurs, we may not have the emotional resilience to withstand the emotional stress and we fall into depression.

What to do?

Making peace with the past and learning to accept yourself exactly how you are, are the keys to deal with grief, disappointment, and loss, all of which are a normal part of life.

Know yourself, spend time going over the past, forgive people and yourself for their shortcomings, and make amends either directly to the people or write letters you do not send. As the Greek philosopher Epictetus said, 'It is not things in themselves that trouble us but our opinion of things'.

Every year 20–25% of adults will have a bout of depression; over a lifetime, this figure rises to 40%.[76] Mental illness is increasing as we become more isolated (see the chapter on Connection); women and poor people suffer more depression, and both groups suffer twice the reported levels of depression. The WHO suggests that in 2030 depression will come only after AIDS in affecting health.

Several things help with depression, meditation, exercise, yoga especially, gentle herbal remedies, talking to others (Samaritans, Age Concern, etc.) and finding a new purpose in this stage of your life.

Grief

Grief is part of ageing: we leave our careers and the camaraderie of workmates, illness may restrict our activities and isolate us, our children leave home, and we lose friends and loved ones; all these losses have a cumulative effect. Grief, then, increasingly becomes part of our experience. The sharp grief of bereavement is the hardest to bear, particularly if the death was unexpected.

Cariad Lloyd's podcast Griefcast[77] has interviewed many grieving people and is well worth a listen for perspectives on grief and being with the bereaved. To summarise: when dealing with the bereaved, you will get it wrong, as each person's grief is unique, and what is helpful for one person is not necessarily helpful for someone else.

Offer practical help: bring food, do the washing up, help with legal issues—Lloyd calls this 'sadmin', which is brilliant. Don't ask what they need; they may not know. Grief can be very overwhelming, so be proactive; you know them and which areas of life they find difficult, practical/emotional/bureaucratic so offer help with that. They might want just to talk, or cry or rage; you don't have to do anything but listen. Avoid asking them how they are as they probably won't know. The generic 'sorry for your loss' can be an irritant. Keep in touch, and send short messages, cards, notes, and texts. They may be ignored at the time, and replying may be too difficult, but they will be remembered fondly later. You can't fix grief, but you can show you care.

Grief comes in all guises. People may look OK, but they may prefer to hide their pain in public to get a respite from the misery. Suicide or violent death brings grief as well as trauma and is particularly hard to deal with. The shame of suicide still remains, and sometimes loved ones feel guilt for not knowing or acting to prevent it. The key is to concentrate on the person who died, not their manner of passing.

There will be trigger times, Christmas, birthdays, anniversary of the death, and even though the person may seem fine it will hurt at these times. Anticipatory grief can be experienced before the person dies, especially with dementia or a lingering terminal diagnosis, and so the grieving process can begin long before their actual death. This does not necessarily mean people won't grieve when death finally occurs; dying is still a shock.

Elizabeth Kubler-Ross, who wrote the seminal book on grief, said,

> The most beautiful people we have known are those who have known defeat, known suffering, known struggle, known loss, and have found their way out of those depths.

Grief is awful, we never get over our loss, but we can find a way through.

Treatment of anxiety or depression is complex, and if it is severe, it is best to consult a health practitioner. But there are lots of things we can do to treat our mood. Sleep, diet, exercise, meditation, Bach Flower, and herbal remedies.

Herbal remedies

Herbal medicine comes into its own with the nervous system. We have many helpful remedies to heal the nervous system and rebalance mood (see Materia Medica for details).

Milky oats and oat straw (*Avena sativa*) are nutritive to the nervous system and the brain. In any issues with the nervous system and the brain, this is the first remedy to build up, heal and soothe.

- Rosemary: stimulates the brain, great for low mood, brain fog and increasing cognitive function.
- Lavender: relaxing to the brain and nervous system, an excellent remedy for anxiety, irritability, insomnia, and panic attacks.
- Skullcap: another nervous system tropho-restorative, which calms anxious, panicky thoughts, and light sleeping due to anxiety and stress.
- Melissa: an excellent remedy for depression and low mood.
- Rose: used for sadness, grief, and shock to the heart.
- Linden blossom: a wonderful relaxing, soothing calming herb which makes a very pleasant tea.
- Violet: useful for sadness; it is soothing and mood-elevating.
- Hops: a bitter sedative for insomnia and acute stress.
- Vervain: another bitter nervine which strengthens and builds up resilience in the nervous system.

Supplements for brain health include Omega 3 fats, zinc, B12, Vitamin E, magnesium, and iron if can't eat well. Or fish oils and multivitamins. Particular foods which support brain health, (in order) are oysters, clams, mussels, watercress, leafy green rainbow vegetables, and grass-fed red meats.

Brain health issues that affect your mind are not necessarily mental illnesses; they may be biological issues affecting the brain. Outcomes in mental health are no better than they were in the 1950s, while their incidence has risen exponentially. This may be attributed the lifestyle changes since then, diet, stress, TV and social media, and pollution. Some psychological illnesses may be primarily a brain problem which subsequently affects the mind and the emotions.

When looking at the brain, we need to consider both psychology and physiology. The state of the physical brain or hardware, and the psychological functions of the brain, how you think (software). The psychological includes what you read, watch, and listen to, and your social circle, because we become like the people we mix with think of this as your 'network connection', to continue the computer analogy. There is also your 'spiritual circle' where we find meaning and purpose in our lives. Therapy can help here also self-hypnosis, affirmations, support groups like Men Without Masks and Sister Circles, herbs, and Bach flower remedies and also online programmes 'everyday bliss' on www.mindvalley.com.

Obesity

Obesity and the size and function of the brain are inversely related: the fatter you are, the more your brain shrinks. Body fat is not innocuous; it increases inflammation, it stores toxins, it takes healthy hormones, and turns them into unhealthy cancer-producing hormones forms of oestrogen. Twenty-five per cent of brain membranes are made from Omega 3, so deficiency means brain doesn't function well (see Thinking).

Brain fog

Brain fog, where the mind is dull and cannot concentrate or think is believed to be connected to gut fermentation.[78]

Fermentation of the gut, where there is bloating and lots of gas, has been called 'the auto-brewery syndrome', where the gut makes its own alcohol from the yeast and sugars which are eaten. This internal fermentation produces a mould (cdifficile) wrongly diagnosed as a condition and not the symptom it is.

The statistics on mental health disease are in themselves depressing and anxiety-producing. It is estimated that depression affects 22% of men and 25% of women over 65 years of age. These statistics relate to reported cases, and it is likely the figures are much higher in reality.

What neuroscience has shown is that you are not stuck with the brain you have (see Thinking). Brain cells don't age; it's the blood vessels in the brain that age, so anything which damages your blood flow damages your brain. So, stimulating the circulation to the brain is important. Herbs such as ginger, ginkgo, pepper, and rosemary stimulate blood flow to the brain, as does exercise especially complex physical movements such as Tai Chi dance.

For particular mood states, herbal medicine works well with the Bach flower remedies (see Materia Medica). They range from acute states like shock and grief, to longstanding conditions like despair or anxiety. They work very well, but patience is needed; it takes time to reverse conditions which have been around for years.

Do not stop taking any medications suddenly. Always seek advice from your doctor or health practitioner—withdrawal symptoms can be alarming, go gently and be kind to yourself

To sum up, for a healthy brain and good mood[79] follow the recommendations in previous chapters. Reduce inflammation in the body through diet, rest, herbal medicine, and exercise. Deal with leaky gut, blood glucose, and low Omega 3 levels. (See the chapter on Fun for ideas on how to use your brain.)

Genetics can be turned on by behaviour (see Thinking: Methylation). There is some research that head trauma may be associated with mental illness (sports injuries, accidents, etc.). Cranial osteopathy which gently manipulates the bones of the skull, can help with this. Toxins of all types affect the blood-rich brain, which soaks up chemicals in our food and in our environment (see Action). It is worthwhile to have a look at what chemicals you come in contact with, especially if your symptoms have come on recently.

New research has shown a link between dementia and inflammation in the gums.[80] They are not sure of the mechanism, but bacteria from gum disease have been found in the brains of dementia sufferers (see recipes for gum health mixtures).

Dr Rahul Jandial[81] gives his checklist for a healthy brain. He sees it as a garden.

1. Nourish: the brain needs nutrients. Eat good food and avoid the insulin response. Make subtle but important changes in your diet, cut out red meat, and HPFs, and add in the Mediterranean diet.
2. Irrigation: The brain has its own pharmacy. For optimal health, the brain needs a good blood supply. Exercise, especially strength training, naturally increases the blood flow to the brain which bathes the brain with BDNF (brain-derived neurotropic factor). The brain loves any kind of inversion (downward dog or headstand in yoga). So, sit less, walk, stand and move more.
3. Rest: fast at least 16 hours one day a week, e.g. 8 pm to 12 pm the next day, i.e. missing breakfast, to give the brain time to repair, and sleep well and deeply.
4. Oxygen and calm: do five minutes of deep breathing three times a day for three minutes. This creates Alpha states in the brain.

5. Read new content for the mind: Be creative: leave a pen next to your bed for those creative thoughts. The best workout is to learn languages or music. The act of learning stretches those parts which have become dormant. Don't have to master it; the benefit comes from trying. Learning to play music builds the greatest connections between the left and right brain and puts you into flow states (increases Alpha states).

6. Try to find happiness, or at least contentment and gratitude: depression and anxiety make changes to the brain. Social connections are important to brain health, and develop or nourish your local networks.

CHAPTER 6

Connection

We are what we feel, and our emotions play a very important role in our overall health and certainly in how we age.

> Kindness—something done with the aim of benefiting someone else.

Kindness is the bedrock of human relationships. Recognise the kindness you see in your world. Behaving kindly brings both emotional and physical benefits and is a buffer against burnout and stress. Kindness brings happiness and can help us to live longer. One of the biggest obstacles to being kind to others is the fear that is their kindness might be misinterpreted: people are afraid of looking stupid among strangers.

You may consider keeping a Kindness Journal and recording three acts of kindness you performed at the end of each day. Whatever we focus on increases. If you focus on kind acts, you will be looking for them and showing your mind it is something you value. Your mind, being the obedient servant it is, will look out for kindness in your daily activities and re-enforce the existence of kindness in your life. This will give you a feeling of pleasure and wellbeing (that dopamine response). As a consequence, you will be alert to potential acts of kindness you could perform and offer more acts of kindness spontaneously (the amygdala again) throughout the day, which will make you happier.

People with social anxiety and introverts are best to start slowly, and perform acts of kindness to people they know, not forgetting to perform acts of kindness to themselves, as self-compassion is also kindness. Examples of kindness include:

Speaking to strangers: a smile or a simple 'How are you' or 'Thank you' can make someone's day. Be safe, of course, there are a few people who see kindness as a weakness to exploit.

Forgiveness: instead of nursing a grudge, let it go, directly to the person or in your heart. Bitterness and resentment only harm us, don't let whatever happened in the past poison your life today. We are all flawed human beings; if someone has behaved badly, it reflects on them and their pain. Of course, some people will use apologies to hurt again, which is why it can sometimes be better to forgive silently and internally.

Helping someone: if someone is struggling and you can help, reach out to them. Sometimes people refuse; again, don't take this to heart; it is their problem not yours, be open-hearted. Most people are good in my experience and will be incredibly grateful for a helping hand.

Inclusion: if someone is being left out, intentionally or unconsciously, reach out to them. It's easy if you're an insider to welcome someone to the group. The feeling of being excluded is very painful; we have all experienced it, be kind to the stranger.

Listening: it is rare that we are listened to, really listened to, without the other person formulating a response. Being heard is such a deep, healing experience, which is why we have helplines and therapists who are trained in 'active listening', which does not judge or offer advice, but simply allows the space for the other person to speak and really be heard.

Volunteering, donations: give away what you no longer need to charity shops, or to freecycle and freegle. Give your time in your community; it will make you feel good about yourself and contributes to longevity.

Random acts of kindness: Think of five kind things to do one day a week (concentration gives bigger rewards) or perform random acts of kindness (indiscriminate altruism) as you go through your day. The brain rewards us when we are kind (oxytocin).

Being kind builds relationships and relationships help us to survive.

However, tainted altruism which are kindnesses performed for effect stems from inauthenticity. This is similar to virtue signalling, which is seen a lot on social media. If you don't mean it, don't do it.

In my experience, most people want to be kind; they often are not sure how it will be received by strangers. During the COVID-19 pandemic, I believe we reconnected with kindness in our communities; when the chips are down, we all know what matters: connection, community and caring for others. Certainly, we understood more than ever the importance of those people who quietly go about their work keeping our lives on track, the lorry drivers delivering food, transport workers, healthcare workers, street cleaners, shopworkers, etc. We understood that money only takes us so far: what we need as humans is contact, other people and their kindness, both to survive and for our mental health.

Giving gifts benefits the giver more than to the recipient. Even recalling a kind act makes you feel better; we can lift heavier weights after thinking of a kindness we performed to someone. A study[82] showed that performing acts of kindness increased feelings of wellbeing. The measured effects were similar to the effects of gratitude, mindfulness, and positive thinking. The study concluded that kindness increases wellbeing. People who helped others because of altruism were found to live longer than those who did not act in this way. Conversely, if kindness to others was motivated by selfish motives (tainted altruism), the health benefit was not seen. The message is to be transparent, be fair, be authentic, and be honest. Be true to yourself, be in alignment so that your outer behaviour is congruent with your values.

Generosity research

Research on the connection between generosity and happiness[83] found that participants who spent money on other people reported greater levels of happiness than those who spent money on themselves over a four-week period. Generous decisions engage the temporo-parietal junction (TPJ) in the brain and increase the connection between the TPJ and ventral striatum. Importantly, striatal activity during generous decisions is directly related to changes in happiness. These results demonstrate that top-down control of striatal activity plays a fundamental role in linking generosity with happiness.

Pro-social behaviour (being a force for good in your community) depends on empathy towards others and has deep social roots. The feel-good, do-good phenomenon of pro-social behaviour makes us feel useful and more connected to our neighbourhood. We feel happier in our homes and with our families. Spontaneous acts of kindness, such as helping a stranger, create more happiness than orderly acts, like supporting charities. Gratitude fosters pro-social behaviour. When we are aware of how blessed we are, even if your life has its challenges, we are more open-hearted towards others who are less fortunate. My experience of working as a volunteer at The Samaritans, was that I felt incredibly grateful for the life I had, when I heard about other people's struggles. Interestingly, reading novels increases our empathy as fiction allows us to experience the lives and battles of other people. Anxiety and depression reduce pro-social behaviour as we tend to become more isolated, which in turn increases anxiety and depression. Social anxiety can be better managed if kindness is woven into everyday life.

Of course, like most things, compassion begins at home with self-compassion. We often say things to ourselves we would never dream of saying to another person. Be kind to yourself; you are doing your best.

A *Guardian* article gave a list of good deeds which always make us happy.[84] It's a great article. Among the suggestions were befriending, helping children's reading skills, fostering an animal, mentoring, and buddy schemes. The possibilities are endless; if you don't want to join a group, litter pick in parks and beaches, do guerrilla gardening by planting flowers in public spaces, help out in homeless shelters or street feeding projects.

Compassion

Dr Julian Abel, a palliative care consultant and joint leader of the Frome project,[85] believes compassion is more powerful than medication.[86]

There are four reasons why compassion is powerful.

Compassion builds social relationships. Many studies show social relationships have a more profound effect on health[87] than any other factor, including stopping smoking, diet, and exercise. Social interaction helps us live longer; it's embedded in our biochemistry and biology. Loneliness increases your chance of dying early by about 30%.[88]

Oxytocin (the hormone associated with compassion), the so-called 'socialising hormone', has receptors all over the body. There would not be so many receptors unless it had an evolutionary advantage, and it does. We survive by being compassionate and being kind. As a species, our existence is due to 'survival of the kindest' rather than 'survival of the fittest'. The Compassionate Community Programme in Frome saw emergency admissions drop by over 30% at a time when they were increasing everywhere else. Because they focused on the social isolation of the patients who used the most resources (medication, hospital visits, GP visits). No other intervention has had this astonishing result.

The compassionate Frome project[89]

Launched in 2013 by Dr Helen Kingston at the Frome Medical Practice who identified that helping patients who were isolated and lonely had a positive impact on their health. These interventions reduced hospital admissions by 30%, a figure unparalleled in medicine. Dr Kingston identified the people who used most of the resources at her practice (the 20% who used 80%) and made them the focus of the study.

She employed 'health connectors' who created a holistic package of health interventions for these patients, while 'volunteer community connectors' delivered personalised support, which ranged from benefit advice, help with shopping, debt advice, and home improvements. Community involvement was encouraged through a variety of groups like, men's sheds, walking groups, choirs, book clubs, etc. A local directory of over 400 local care providers and volunteers was collected, to re-connect people. The web directory was for everyone, and the practice trained people how to access this information. Dr Kingston realised that her GP practice was only one of a whole raft of interventions available to improve wellbeing. And although going to the GP may have been the first step when a person feels unwell, the centre developed many other resources which could be used other than prescribing drugs. They trained over 700 community connectors, people listening out for others, often those who had been helped themselves by the project. They were 'people helping people' who were trained in motivational interviewing and who worked 1:1 with people. From the GP's perspective, they were able to direct people to places where they could address their underlying issues and get the correct support.

Our social interactions may be fleeing, but they are still valuable: chatting to the till operator, the bus driver or postman, and saying hello to your neighbours. These heart-warming experiences and day-to-day interactions increase the oxytocin secreted in your body and your blood pressure drops. Studies show a 50% increased likelihood of survival for participants with stronger social relationships. This finding remained consistent across age, sex, initial health status, cause of death, and follow-up period, and the association was strongest for complex measures of social integration and lowest for living alone.[90] Love, laughter, and friendship keep us healthy.

Pain is also influenced by mood and emotions. Dr Julian Abel,[91] a consultant in palliative (end-of-life) care, says pain can never be entirely managed through drugs; the mental state of the patient has a massive effect. In his experience, if you work with the emotions and issues around loved ones, a similar painkilling effect is seen. If people are feeling loved and secure, their anxiety reduces, their pain levels go down, then oxytocin is produced as well as endorphins (morphine-like compounds which we naturally produce) which dull the pain. Your biochemistry, physiology, and biology change when you have close social connections.

Each of us can be a little more compassionate; once you start, you will never stop. The rewards are so brilliant. Compassion leads to friendship, love, and laughter. We are already compassionate; devote some time to appreciate your compassion. It will help you live a long and happy life.

How can you apply this in your life?

Reaching out, tell loved ones you love them, making new connections, and renewing old friendships, take small steps.

CHAPTER 7

Fun

As important as community, is pleasure. My experience of ageing is re-defining what is fun for me. It won't be what it looked like ten years ago, or 20 years ago, but spend a little time working out what makes your heart sing; that is my definition of fun. There is a Japanese word, *ikigai*, which means 'reason to get up in the morning'. When we are working less, or at least working less towards certain goals, we may need to re-configure what our *ikigai* is now.

Ikigai comes at the confluence of …

- That which you love: passion/mission.
- That which you are good at: passion/profession.
- That which the world needs: mission/vocation.
- That which you can be paid for: vocation/profession.

I understand work may not be central as we age, but a recent series of articles in the *Guardian* newspaper 'Life after sixty'[92] interviewed men and women who have reinvented themselves in later life. Often these stories cover people who have always wanted to do something, and find themselves in their 60s saying, 'It's now or never'. People have begun marathon running, teaching cookery, becoming an actor, joining a band, training as a hospice nurse, learning to ride a motorbike, learning to swim, becoming an artist, and adventure cycling. If you are needing some inspiration, do look up the article.

Many people report that there is a second flowering of career after 60. For the reasons above, we are freer than we have been in recent years, probably as free as when we were young. Sometimes, we have more resources to invest in our interests, and certainly, we usually have more time, if not more energy.

Contentment

Christopher Boyce,[93] behavioural scientist, has studied happiness, and these are his conclusions:

Go deep: Money, above a certain level (basic needs met), does not bring happiness; stuff doesn't bring happiness after a certain level, remember the joy of something you bought that you saved up for as a child, now when we buy things that joy is often absent or diminished. What is important is connection, purpose, and hope.

Goals: have goals, a direction, or a roadmap but be prepared to let your goals change. Indeed, it has been shown achieving goals can be depressing. The classic let-down of achieving your aims leaves you with depression and anxiety. What now? So, immerse yourself in the journey toward your goals, but remain flexible; it may be there are forks in the road which may give you greater joy than continuing towards a goal.

Accept help: allow others to help; people love to be useful. Remain open to others, accept their input with grace.

Know you have survived several crises in your life: You made it through, and you are here now reading this. You have great inner strength and resilience. Acknowledge this.

Take time to smell the roses or watch the stars: Be here now and enjoy this moment. You are alive; not everyone has this gift, so make it special.

Reading

We may have lost the habit of reading books, but recent research has shown how reading, fiction or non-fiction, is associated with longevity and better health.[94] People who read books, not magazines or newspapers, lived on average two years longer than their non-reading peers when other variables such as race, sex, and income were considered. The effects were long-lasting; after 12 years, they had a 20% drop in mortality compared with non-readers. This is a huge result. The study (University of Michigan) measured 3,645 people, so it was a large group. It did not seem to matter how much reading was done, except that it was whole books, not articles, that were read. Reading has two effects on the brain (cognitive outcomes): first, it promotes 'deep reading', which is a slow process where the reader becomes immersed in the book (rather than the skim reading we do on websites/newspapers, etc.). The reader holds what is currently being read, with what was previously read, and weaves them into the narrative they are following, makes connections with what they already know of the world and asks questions about what they have read, improving vocabulary, critical thinking, reasoning, and concentration are all improved.

Second, books promote empathy, social perception, and emotional intelligence, all of which are linked to improving survival rates.[95] This may be due to reduced stress levels and a feeling of connection with society, and using the brain creatively. These effects were found to be independent of gender, educational achievement, and income. Most people who read books and read fiction (87%); reading a chapter a day (30 minutes reading time) showed this cognitive advantage, which was long-lasting. Libraries are wonderful resources for a whole variety of books.

Which books to read? Non-fiction can teach us lots of facts, but you can easily chapter-hop to subjects you are interested in.

Conversely, reading fiction means you have to hold the whole narrative in your head as you read the story, remember details as you go along and empathise with the character and follow the plot. One of the signs of early dementia is that people often stop reading novels, as they cannot follow the story easily.[96]

Music

Research has shown that music has a positive effect on our wellbeing.[97] Music is universal among all cultures. Darwin believed music was created to attract partners; since his day, there have been many theories about why we humans make music and what it does to our bio-psycho-social-spiritual lives. Musicality (the ability to create and perceive music) bonds us together socially. Any concert, gig or music festival goer will attest to the intense shared experience of the audience, who may have little in common except for their love of the music.

Music creates social bonding, as we are beings who live in groups; music is psychologically and biologically central to our reproduction and survival as a species: enhanced predator protection, cooperative child rearing, collaborative foraging, defence of our territory all work better in groups, think neighbourhood watch groups, cooperatives, childcare groups, special interest groups, etc.

We are group animals, however introverted any individual is, and we hunt (or supermarket forage) and protect ourselves and our loved ones in groups. Music forges and strengthens relationships within a group by harmonising emotions, moods, and the perspectives of two or more people. Music can do this where language is less able to express feelings. A larger group of music lovers experiences this social bonding compared to the more intimate social bonding, such as cooking meals, joint activities, etc. In short, we come together through music. Scientists call this 'identity fusion'. This is why group songs are so powerful; national anthems, rousing songs (Land of Hope and Glory), football chants, political songs (Oh Jeremy Corbyn at Glastonbury in 2017), Westminster Cathedral, on Christmas Eve, the solo 'Once in Royal David's City', Italians singing from their balconies during the lockdowns of 2020, humans are evolved to be musical. Music evokes intense emotions as it brings us together; music is often associated with physical movements such as hand clapping, foot taping, and dance, all of which stimulate the brain, bring pleasure, and are great exercise. There are many opportunities to experience music in groups, from drumming workshops to lunchtime classical concerts, choirs, gigs, and dance classes. We may have lost the habit of going to public music events as we have grown older, but music has a great deal to offer to keep us connected to both our hearts and our community.

Dancing

As we grow older, we tend to let go of our enjoyment (if we had it) of moving our bodies to music. Like music, dancing is something found in all cultures; dancing is ingrained in human behaviour (see Move on the cognitive benefits of dancing). Moving together in rhythm, such as group dancing, or couple dancing, the brainwaves of the dancers begin to synchronise.[98] This is surely an incentive to dance with loved ones if one were needed. Research has found that dancing and listening to music have a positive effect on mood (it makes you happy) and increases creativity.[99] Dancing releases endorphins (nature's happy hormones) which relieve anxiety and depression.

Treats

Ageing gracefully does not have to be a 'hairshirt' experience. We can enjoy many things while building resilience and health.

Red wine

Red wine contains resveratrol, an antioxidant also found in peanuts, blueberries, raspberries, and mulberries. Preliminary research has shown a variety of benefits,[100] including, anti-obesity, cardioprotective, neuroprotective, antitumor, antidiabetic, antioxidants, anti-age effects, and on glucose metabolism. However, the quantities required to have these effects cannot be found in foods. Drinking a glass of red wine daily may not show these therapeutic benefits, but it is a good alcohol to drink, a neat treat. Red wine with chocolate has double the effect!

Chocolate

Chocolate contains compounds which have been found to improve mood or reduce negative mood states. It also shows an improvement in cognitive function, although it was not clear whether the pleasure in eating the chocolate gave this effect or the compounds found in dark chocolate. Chocolate's active constituents are methylxanthines, caffeine, and theobromine, which may have effects similar to caffeine, and also flavonoids. High levels of flavonoids are also found in green tea, grapes, red wine, and apples.[101]

Coffee

Hurray, finally we know how good coffee is for you! Not too much, but a little has many benefits for health. These benefits depend on how much the coffee is roasted; the lower the roast, the more benefit. For example, coffee in Italy has less chlorogenic acid (the beneficial compound) than in Spain, which lightly roasts its coffee. Instant coffee contains varying amounts depending on how it is processed.[102] Among the health benefits of coffee are lowering blood pressure,[103] improving glucose regulation[104] and improving cardiovascular health.[105]

Sex[106]

Sex is a normal human activity, with many health benefits. Recent research by OnePoll[107] looked at the sex lives of 1,200 people aged 60 and above. Forty-eight per cent felt more confident in their sexual relationships than ever before, with 19% feeling more confident than when they were younger. Thirty-nine per cent said that sex continues to be an important part of their relationships, while 45% said they felt more relaxed about sex and intimacy than previously. What was depressing was that 53% believed that society had a negative view of older people enjoying sex and intimacy.

Biologically, post-menopause the drop in oestrogen levels affects the vaginal tissues by making them less flexible and reducing lubrication. This might cause issues around intercourse (vaginismus) and irritation of the vulva and vagina. Vaginal lubricants[108] can help here and in extremis HRT creams when the pain is severe and unremitting. Pelvic floor exercises have been shown to help[109] also using pessaries made from fennel and sea buckthorn.[110]

The science of sex and love is fascinating. When you fall in love, and see the face of your beloved, you experience a dopamine surge. Dr Helen Fisher measured the brains of people in love with an MRI.[111] Falling in love is indeed like an addiction (see Thinking on dopamine and the brain), causing euphoria and dependency.[112] As dopamine rises so does testosterone, which fuels sexual feelings in both men and women. Dopamine also depresses serotonin. Low serotonin levels are found in both people with obsessive-compulsive disorders and people in love, which may explain the obsession of the lover.

The lovers' brains were retested after seven months, and the dopamine levels had returned to normal; that mad, obsessive phase was over, or the temporary insanity had passed. What followed was the settling in of the 'married' phase of the relationship. The relationship then becomes warm, not hot, where affection, security, trust, and love dominate. These feelings are mediated by oxytocin and vasopressin, which are produced in the reproductive organs and the hypothalamus, which is the seat of the emotions which foster the connection and closeness of intimate sex rather than passion. So how to rekindle the fire and increase those dopamine levels?

Novelty—get away from the everyday; they are not called romantic getaways for nothing. Researchers found couples' shared participation in novel and challenging activities, if not overly stressful, may promote increases in romantic love as the reward-value associated with the experience becomes associated with the relationship'.[113]

Have fun. Dopamine is increased when we laugh. Try new tricks and techniques; boredom is the enemy of passion. While novelty can spice up your love life.

Couples who have regular sex feel more connected to their partner and rate their relationship happiness much higher than couples who don't. Sex and intimacy make us happy, and fosters closeness; why on earth would we want to let sex or intimacy disappear from our lives?

Tracey Cox, author of *Great Sex Starts after Fifty*. Wrote how surprised she was when writing the book, how few long-established couples talked about sex, what they liked, what they wanted to try out and what was a turn-off.[114] She gives hints on how to introduce the subject sensitively and kindly.

TV

Future generations will look back on TV as the lead in the water pipes that slowly drove the Romans mad.

Kurt Vonnegut

I have to admit I am a fervid opponent of TV watching and have been so all my adult life. Science has now given fuel to my aversion to fire.[115] Watching TV is associated with increased mortality rates. The figures are startling, watching more than three hours of TV daily is associated with an increased mortality due to all causes 12%, and for each additional hour of watching TV mortality risks increased by 4%. The researchers looked at whether this was due to inactivity, but those who were physically active had the same outcomes. The advertising of unhealthy food and drinks or risky behaviours, such as gambling, had some effect, as people were more likely to order in HPF after seeing it advertised. The researchers suggest it was the content of the TV programmes had an effect.

The study excluded people who were unwell, as sick people often watch more TV when they are recovering. It is well known that people who watch a lot of TV are more likely to be obese, smoke, have a sedentary lifestyle, have poor diets, have lower educational attainment, and have lower social capital (they do not interact with the community, volunteer, or socialise). TV watchers have higher rates of cardiovascular disease; this was previously believed to be due to the unhealthy choices mentioned above.

However, it turns out that it is the emotional experience of TV watching that causes the harm. This was a study carried out over 30 years, from 1978–2008, in the US. Exposure to violent images increases stress in the autonomic system (fight-or-flight mechanism; see digestion for a discussion of cortisol in health). The researchers believed the brain experiences this watched violence as real threats and that prolonged viewing of violent content increases the stress response with all its concomitant health risks.

TV watching also impacts on feelings of happiness or depression. Those who watched more TV felt less trusting of others, felt afraid in their neighbourhood, experienced less general happiness, felt less supported by people, and the government, religion, science, and their community. They felt like victims of life and its randomness, had less trust and overall satisfaction with their life.

Those who watched TV for less than three hours a day did not show these effects or increased mortality. The results were consistent between 1978 and 2008, suggesting it was not increased HPFs or decreased physical activity which were responsible (as HPFs were rare in 1978 and people were more active overall). Advertising (in the US) for harmful products (guns?) was less common in 2008 than in 1978. However, TV content has arguably become more violent, nightly news, murder shows which increase anxiety, feelings of helplessness, anger, and rage at other people the media blames for our ills (immigrants, women, black people, Muslims, etc.) all of which increase the feeling of impotent rage and its consequent physiological effects.

One interesting finding was there was less interpersonal trust and trust in the US and its institutions in those who watched three hours or more TV. These people felt more isolated and afraid. There was no correlation between socio-economic class; this effect was seen across the board. Social capital is the best indicator of longevity. Turn off that TV and meet real people who share your interests.

In this chapter, we have discussed ways of having fun; I'm sure you can think of others …

CHAPTER 8

Checking out

> Death is not extinguishing the light, but putting out
> the lamp because the dawn has come.
>
> Rabindranath Tagore

A good death, a death with dignity, can happen when the death is aligned with the personal values of the dying person. A good death happens when symptoms, especially pain, are controlled and when patients and family recognise death as a sacred experience which can be treasured. Death with dignity can bring healing to the dying person and their loved ones. There can be true closure and celebration of a life well lived.

Dr Julian Abel, a consultant in palliative care,[116] has spoken to thousands of dying people. He asked what mattered to them as they lay in hospital beds. People spoke of feeling a diminished sense of self because their illness meant they were no longer able to do the things that had previously brought them happiness. In our culture, we are led to believe acquisition is the route to happiness. When we are dying, we realise that what is really important is the love we experience from the people around us, their care, and friendship. We value people for their character, their kindness and consistency.

Although the body begins to fail, our ability to be loving and kind remains. Even if we are immobile, we can still give love and be a friend by forgiving those who have hurt us, apologising to those we have let down, in other words, putting our 'emotional affairs in order'. Dr Abel saw that those who died peacefully were usually satisfied by how their lives had been and had loving friends and family. People loved them for who they were and not because of what they did or owned. These people prioritised their relationships, and they were kind and compassionate people (see Happiness).

These ideas, of course, are best implemented before we become ill, but a good reminder of the important things in life.

Five top deathbed wishes[117]

This comes from a hospice nurse who has sat at the bedside of many, many dying people.

1. I wish I'd had the courage to live a life true to myself, not the life others expected of me.

    This was the most common regret of all. When people realise that their life is almost over and look back clearly on it, it is easy to see how many dreams have gone unfulfilled. Most people have had not honoured even half of their dreams and had to die knowing that it was due to choices they had made, or not made. It is very important to try and honour at least some of your dreams along the way. From the moment that you lose your health, it is too late. Health brings a freedom very few realise, until they no longer have it.

2. I wish I hadn't worked so hard.

    This came from every male patient that I nursed. They missed their children's youth and their partner's companionship. Women also spoke of this regret. But as most were from an older generation, many of the female patients had not been breadwinners. All of the men I nursed deeply regretted spending so much of their lives on the treadmill of a work existence.

By simplifying your lifestyle and making conscious choices along the way, it is possible to not need the income that you think you do. And by creating more space in your life, you become happier and more open to new opportunities, ones more suited to your new lifestyle.

3. I wish I'd had the courage to express my feelings.

Many people suppressed their feelings in order to keep peace with others. As a result, they settled for a mediocre existence and never became who they were truly capable of becoming. Many developed illnesses relating to the bitterness and resentment they carried as a result.

We cannot control the reactions of others. However, although people may initially react when you change the way you are by speaking honestly, in the end it raises the relationship to a whole new and healthier level. Either that or it releases the unhealthy relationship from your life. Either way, you win.

4. I wish I had stayed in touch with my friends.

Often, they would not truly realise the full benefits of old friends until their dying weeks, and it was not always possible to track them down. Many had become so caught up in their own lives that they had let golden friendships slip by over the years. There were many deep regrets about not giving friendships the time and effort that they deserved. Everyone misses their friends when they are dying.

It is common for anyone with a busy lifestyle to let friendships slip. But when you are faced with your approaching death, the physical details of life fall away. People do want to get their financial affairs in order if possible. But it is not money or status that holds the true importance for them. They want to get things in order more for the benefit of those they love. Usually, though, they are too ill and weary to ever manage this task. It is all comes down to love and relationships in the end. That is all that remains in the final weeks, love, and relationships.

5. I wish that I had let myself be happier.

This is a surprisingly common one. Many did not realise until the end that happiness was a choice. They had stayed stuck in old patterns and habits. The so-called 'comfort' of familiarity overflowed into their emotions, as well as their physical lives. Fear of change had them pretending to others, and to their selves, that they were content. When deep within, they longed to laugh properly and have silliness in their life again.

When you are on your deathbed, what others think of you is a long way from your mind. How wonderful to be able to let go and smile again, long before you are dying.

Three women have written seminal books on the care of the dying.[118] Cecily Saunders began the hospice movement in the UK after seeing how badly dying patients were treated in hospitals. Her main focus was on managing pain relief so the person could have a peaceful death. Elizabeth Kubler-Ross saw the same lack of care in the US and wrote her ground-breaking book, *On Death and Dying*, where she described the five-stage model of grief, for patients as they realised their diagnosis was terminal. Felicity Warner wrote *A Safe Journey Home* about the stages of dying and she started Soul Midwives who work with the dying, again so they can have a peaceful, fear-free, death.

Soul midwives

A gentler death, what we all hope for, can be achieved by combining the best care that medicine can provide alongside the subtler methods such as massage, visualisation, breathing techniques, and other holistic ways of calming and soothing.

Felicity Warner, *A Safe Journey Home*, 2011, p. xvii

Death cafes

The first UK Death Cafe was opened in Hackney by Jon Under-
wood and Sue Barsky Reid based on the ideas of sociologist
Bernard Crettaz who opened the first Death Cafe in Switzerland
following his wife's death. At a Death Cafe, people meet to
eat cake, drink tea, and discuss death. Their objective is: 'to
increase awareness of death with a view to helping people
make the most of their (finite) lives'.

A Death Cafe is not a grief support meeting or a counselling
session; it is a neutral space where people can talk freely about
dying. Death Cafes have spread quickly across Europe, North
America, and Australasia. Their popularity shows that people
want to break the taboo of speaking about death and want to
discuss the issues in a non-clinical setting. Lizzy Miles[119] ran
the first Death Cafe in the US and Megan Mooney,[120] who runs
the Death Cafe Facebook page[121] have played a significant
role in Death Cafe's development. Everyone has their own
reasons for getting involved in a Death Cafe. In a video on
their website (see www.deathcafe.org and https://deathcafe.
com/profile/406/), Death Cafe Portland organiser Kate
Brassington explains hers.

Reaction to a terminal diagnosis

In *On Death and Dying* (1969), physician Elizabeth Kubler-Ross
described the process she observed people with a terminal illness went through as they came to terms with their dying.
Her five stages of grief have wrongly been applied to people
who are bereaved, but her original work was with patients
in a hospital who were given a terminal diagnosis and were,
at that time, often ignored by doctors and left to die without
support.

The five stages are not necessarily consecutive and earlier
stages may return as death grows nearer. But they do work in

my experience and can be applied not only to the dying but also to any major life event such as redundancy and divorce.

The first stage is denial: the person believes the diagnosis is wrong, and they avoid people who might counter their beliefs and may therefore become isolated from loved ones. They may try all kinds of therapies before they reach an understanding that death is coming.

The second stage is anger: it is clear denial won't solve the issue, and they want to lash out at carers because 'it's not fair' 'why is this happening to me?' etc., etc. For loved ones and carers, it is important to allow the person to express their anger without taking it personally; it is just a stage and will pass.

The third stage is bargaining: the person will make a deal to stay alive for a wedding or other important occasion, and they may extend their death as they wait for a loved one to travel to see them. This may be hours, days, months and sometimes even years that they hold on.

The fourth stage is depression: resignation and realisation of death occurs, and the person may feel hopeless, refuse to be comforted, and wish to be alone. Again, for carers do try not to deny these feelings and take their behaviour personally. It will pass.

The final stage is acceptance: the person acknowledges they are dying and prepares for it. This is a good time to write out the Death Plan (see below) and speak to a Soul Midwife, visit a Death Cafe, plan the funeral, and reach out to people they wish to see. In this stage, the person becomes calm and peaceful, and there is a freedom in acceptance. The dying person may arrive at acceptance before loved ones, which can cause hurt feelings. Acceptance may also involve amends and reparations needing to be made to loved ones and 'putting one's affairs in order' and releasing and relinquishing the unnecessary in their lives. Carers can listen closely and follow the directions of the dying person at this stage which will bring peace and release to their loved one as their life is put in order.

Assisted dying

Assisted dying[122] is at present illegal in the UK. It was legalised in Oregon in 2017 and is now legal in California, Washington, and other US states. Assisted dying is not assisted suicide and only applies to people who have less than six months to live and who have the mental capacity to make that decision. There is a cooling-off period where people can reflect on their decision, and an assessment by a High Court Judge and/or doctors is made. Only the dying person may do this. This allows them to die peacefully at home rather than travel to a Swiss clinic to fulfil their wishes. Those who do not support assisted dying should not be made to do so (doctors, nurses, etc.) and the act is entirely in the hands of the person who knows there is no chance of recovery and wishes to die with dignity.

Presently, if you travel with a person to Dignitas in Switzerland or help them commit suicide in any way, you may be liable to 14 years in prison in the UK, although the CPS uses discretion in deciding whether to charge carers. There is huge support for this among the general public: 84% of people believe we should have this right and over 44% of people would break the law to help a loved one.[123] Compassion in dying[124] has resources for planning your end-of-life care, including writing a living will outlining treatment opt-outs.

Psychedelics and the end of life

One thing that psychedelics offer us is an opportunity to re-evaluate our lives and make peace with ourselves and others. Psilocybin is illegal in the UK, but clinical trials are happening in Manchester and Kings College London on its use for patients with a terminal diagnosis (see Action for psychedelics).

Care for the dying

Felicity Warner, in *A Safe journey Home* (2011), gives lots of tips on how to care for a dying loved one to make the process of dying as gentle and fear-free as possible. She describes death as, 'a process rather than an event, the gradual unravelling of life a slow and gentle letting go', and 'like a feather taking off in the wind'.[125]

Having experienced many deaths, she considers that people die as they have lived, some peacefully, some raging, some fearful. If the death is a gentle one, it can bring healing to the carer and the loved ones, especially if the death happens at home. Seventy per cent of people want to die at home, but in the UK only 17% manage this.

Fear of dying has increased as death has moved into the hospital. Clinical settings can increase fear and pain, especially if it occurs in an ICU and the person is wired up to machines and the staff is harried, and there is no sense of calm or tenderness. Do listen to this shocking report by ZDogg MD (see https://zdoggmd.com/end-of-life/), who describes a resuscitation of the dying and its effect on the patient. ZDogg MD describes the grim reality of what happens in an ICU resuscitation, how the patient responds and the likely outcome.

A do not resuscitate (DNR) order can be added to your medical notes if you do not wish to go through this procedure. ZDogg suggests putting your wishes down clearly and speaking with family members beforehand to make things clear, because in the heat of the moment they may wish to do anything to prevent you from dying.

A death at home can happen with music playing, loved ones near, hands and feet massaged with essential oils, sound baths, favourite music, others keeping vigil, and food prepared and eaten; in other words, death can be a gentle and loving experience.

Death plan

Consider how you wish your death to be and write it down clearly.[126]

- Do you wish loved ones with you, or do you wish to be alone of in a hospice or nursing home?
- What kind of treatment do you wish to have as you begin to die, if any? Pain relief? When do you wish treatment to stop?
- What kind of emotional and spiritual support would you like?
- You have the right to refuse food and drink.
- You may choose to die at your own hand if your life feels intolerable.
- How long do you wish your body to be left before a funeral or cremation?
- How do you wish the body to be prepared (embalming, anointing etc)?
- How do you wish to be buried/cremated?
- What type of funeral do you wish to have, or none?

The purpose of being clear on these questions is that being at ease with the idea of dying allows us to enjoy life and perhaps live in the present.

For the carer

If you don't have loved ones or you don't want them to sit with you, there are Soul Midwives and Death Doulas who can offer this service, to provide nurturing, support, and reassurance and visit the family afterwards to facilitate closure.

As a companion to a dying person, you will try to hear their fears without judgement and listen to them and remind them of all the death they have experienced in their lives, parents, from childhood to adulthood, etc. Often people experience the Dark Night of the Soul as death approaches.[127] It can last for days. The person starts to doubt their belief systems or faith. This stage is linked to the final act of surrender when they must detach from all comforting belief systems and enter the bleak chasm.[128] This is a sign the ego is dissolving and can be a painful, frightening process. When the person surrenders to the darkness, their energy shifts from fear to enlightenment. A useful meditation is imagining quietly slipping between two worlds without pain and being surrounded by love. Or imagining scenarios of your death as peaceful, in a garden, in sleep, gently exhaling.[129] Sometimes it is helpful to charge up a talisman, jewellery, or a crystal for them to carry through the process to give them courage.

Breathing techniques can be helpful if there is panic. The carer can mirror their breathing and then take longer and longer breaths; the patient will then begin to calm down. Working with psychedelics on receipt of a terminal diagnosis may help to reconcile to death (see Action).

Sitting with the dying is easier when there is a bond of trust and empathy. A quick way to build trust and a heart-soul connection is to hold their feet or massage their feet. This flesh-to-flesh contact or loving touch[130] is very soothing and healing. Reiki or Spiritual Healing is also helpful here. Sometimes, direct touch is too much, so gently blow or hover above their feet and send loving energy to them. Anointing is an ancient practice used to send the dying peacefully away[131] with sacred oils.[132] Anoint the palms and soles of the feet, the crown chakra and the heart chakra to help the spirit separate from the body. The essential oils of sandalwood, rose, and myrrh are especially helpful.

The senses are enhanced as a person dies, which is why ICUs are not an ideal place to die. The dying react to bright lights, loud noises, and uncomfortable surroundings. As hearing is the final sense to go, speak softly and gently when you are around the dying.

People need to know they have been loved and their lives had meaning. It may be helpful to recount happy memories, look at old photos, or tell family stories. Be sure to speak their name often.

Smell is important (it is mediated by the limbic system). Fragrances inhaled by the left nostril are more likely to be perceived as positive. Place oil burners or incense on that side. Aromas trigger memory, which may recall happy times. Vanilla is a favourite smell as it is the fragrance of mother's milk. Scented candles, spritzing the bedding, burning incense, washing the face and hands with hydrosols like rose water all bring feelings of peace and calm.

As we die, our vision narrows and we only see what is in front of us, so be sure to sit facing the person when you enter the room. Colour influences mood surrounding the dying in gentle, nourishing colours like pink, soft green, and apricot.

Simple tips for vigil as dying begins[133]

Touch them, hold their hands, massage their feet, moisten their eyes with a warm damp cotton wool, use gentle herbal mouth-washes if teeth brushing is too uncomfortable. Check their ears are lying flat, and that they are comfortable. If possible, change the position of the head and shoulders every hour. Use simple breathing techniques to calm and centre both you and the dying person. Learn a simple visualisation when you are sitting, perhaps focusing on the heart or the breath, while they are waiting for pain meds to work. Burn essential oils like sandalwood, geranium, rose, or vanilla to keep the air fresh. If they are in hospital or a hospice, bring bedding or pillows from home to make them comfortable.

Softly singing or saying 'all will be well' is comforting. If you have a spiritual practice, chanting is also helpful. Have dim lights or candlelight, or orange bulbs to create a soothing atmosphere.

If they are dying in a busy household, having a baby alarm in their room is useful so they can be in touch while others are going about their daily lives.

Bring the outside in, put flowers in the room, and have the bed facing a window if possible. Keep the room clean and calm. Change the sheets daily if possible, and add colour and soft blankets, nice music, and have their laptop, radio, torch, candles, etc. nearby.

As dying begins, vigils[134]

The four stages of dying can take weeks or months or can occur instantly with a sudden death or in sleep unexpectedly. Death occurs as each of the Four Elements are withdrawn from the body one by one.

Earth is the first element to go. The person complains of tiredness, aches, and pains; they may be nauseous and repelled by smells, and want all perfumes, candles, oil burners etc., to be removed from their room. Their complexion fades, their face becomes grey and waxy, their strength goes. They may be more tearful and afraid of being alone.

Next, Water departs. Their taste changes, they may refuse foods and drinks they previously liked, it becomes hard to chew, fluid leaves the body through a runny nose, their eyes may water, they may dribble and become incontinent. They can experience a sense of drowning or heaviness like pushing through water, or a sinking sensation.

Then Fire leaves. There may be sudden temperature fluctuations, shivering, burning, and sweating, the lips may crack from dryness and the mouth becomes parched. They may experience nose bleeds, and the hands and feet become cold as warmth leaves the extremities. There may be alternating clarity and confusion, restlessness and apprehension, followed finally by a calm detachment.

Lastly, the Air element leaves the body. The hearing may go, and breathing becomes difficult and erratic with rasping, panting, and missing breaths. These short breaths eventually lead to a final breath as the death rattle comes, and they may cry out while awake or asleep.

When they die, people enter the final active phase, which is both physical, as the body begins to shut down, and spiritual, as out-of-body consciousness expands they may see and hear things others cannot and may have powerful dreams or visions.

There may be rallies or a sudden exit from life. As death grows nearer, they become withdrawn, and their appetite goes. There may be agitation or restlessness; they want to be moved or complain the room is too hot or cold or noisy. There is increased sleep, irregular breathing, and poor wound healing.

As death happens[135] remove all sensory stimulation, switch off the lights and burn white candles to foster an atmosphere of calmness. If there is fear or panic, encourage them to release, and let go, breathe with them to lengthen their breaths. Tell them they are loved and safe. Give them permission to move on and say loved ones are waiting for them on the other side. At the moment of death, the energy in the room may feel like shockwaves; there is a sudden chill, and the atmosphere may be disturbed. Open a window to release the soul.

To ease the passing, the following may be spritzed over the dying or dropped on their head.[136] The Bach flower remedies walnut, honeysuckle, cherry plum, heather, Rescue Remedy and Star of Bethlehem may be helpful. The best gemstones for the dying are quartz, smoky quartz, rose quartz, amethyst, and aquamarine, which can be placed on or around the dying person. This may be a time for chanting, sounding singing bowls, telling ancestral tales, ringing bells or lovingly sharing deep silence. Repeat blessings or prayers or mantras. As you keep vigil, pay full attention, open your heart, remember it is their time, and leave your personal concerns outside the room. Have a simple ritual at the end with candles, incense, or sound.

After death

After death, you may wish to wash the body, anoint it with oils and prepare it for burial, dressing it in meaningful clothes, or grave goods. Light a candle for them. Use this mourning time to grieve and nourish. If the death happened at home, invite people around, eat, drink, and fill the house with love and tenderness.

Care for the carer

Look after yourself as you look after the dying person. People who are ill can suck the energy of carers. Dying people can be angry and manipulative as they process their shadow soul pain; they can project it outwards on to carers and loved ones.[137] The best carers listen to their fear and pain and resist the urge to fix or impose their beliefs on the dying person. Help the dying person to find their own peace and see a wider perspective. Be as non-judgemental as you can by honouring their reality. Offer them unconditional love and be empathetic and compassionate.

As a carer it is important to protect, nourish, and heal yourself. Take time to go into nature, shower after visiting (water washes energy form the body), eat wholesome food, spend time alone in silence, or in blue/white lighting, and do aura cleansing.

After death, open windows in the room and allow the sunlight in. Do wholesome everyday tasks like baking bread, digging the garden, do energetic work on your body, such as Restorative Yoga, and Tai Chi. Bathe in sensual essential oils, and spend time with animals and children who have high, clean energy to recalibrate. Dive into your creativity, which nourishes soul and spirit, sing, swim in the sea or lakes, chanting your name[138] is a way of reclaiming your energy and identity after an intense experience.

What happens when we die?
The Near-Death Experience (NDE)

One way to get a sense of what awaits us on the 'other side' is the study of Near-Death Experiences. Since the 1970s, there has been huge amounts of research on NDE. Partly because of advances in trauma medicine, more people survive conditions which would have previously been fatal. Dr Raymond Moody's ground-breaking book, *Life and After Life* (1975) investigated 150 cases of NDE. Moody and later researchers found patients had similar experiences, whether they were religious previously or not, irrespective of the type of trauma, be it a heart attack, accident, long-awaited death, or suicide.

Understanding the phenomena of NDE can help to allay the fear of dying and also give comfort to the bereaved. Extraordinarily, researchers have now identified another phenomenon, Shared Death Experiences (SDE), where carers, doctors, and nurses have similar experiences at the bedside of a dying person, and some accompany them to the 'after life'.

In the NDE, there is a commonality of experience which includes:

- The body rising upwards as they see the resuscitation happening below.
- They pass through a dark enclosure, 'the tunnel', into a brilliant, white light.
- 'The experience is ineffable and indescribable. Words are inadequate. They say that in the bright light, they feel comfort, joy, peace, and love so intense as to be almost palpable'.[139]
- Spirits of dead loved ones wait to welcome them.
- A hologram of their life flashes before them; they experience it in vivid detail, instantly, and from the viewpoint of others who were present at the events.

For some people, they are suddenly returned to their bodies. Others say they were told to return by one of the spirits as they had things to do. Others were given a choice. Those who chose to return, although the majority would have preferred to stay, came back for someone else, often to raise young children.

Once back, they all said the NDE totally altered their perspective on life. They understood there was an afterlife, and those things they were striving for previously, money, power, fame, etc., became unimportant. They understood that the only thing that was important in life was learning to love.

Biological causes of NDE phenomena have been discounted, especially as medical practitioners and carers began to report their experiences of SDE. SDE experiences included leaving their bodies, and accompanying the dying person as they moved towards the light. Onlookers sometimes described that at the moment of death a bright light filled the room; they heard indescribably beautiful music, saw the deceased's loved ones and, occasionally, were present at the life-review.

Dr Moody[140] suggests these experiences have profound implications for carers as well as solace for the dying. If someone tells you they have experienced SDE, listen to their experience without judgement. Give them the reassurance that thousands of others have had the same experiences and these experiences do not make them 'crazy'; they are not mentally ill. NDEs and SDEs are not rare; it's just there is shame and embarrassment in speaking of them.

Moody's research was replicated by other respected scientists, and the body of evidence has grown and confirmed his findings. Given dying is an intense psycho-spiritual experience for both the patient and carer, the importance of creating a sacred space for the dying is clear. Whether it is at home, in hospital or in a hospice, creating a calm, peaceful and loving atmosphere will make the process of dying easier for everyone.

Death can be an ecstatic experience. Loved ones are waiting for us, all is well, and there is no more fear and pain. Death is something to be welcomed when the time comes.

Grieving

I called this chapter 'Checking out' because I feel that leaving this meat suit is not the end of our story. I very much like Louise Hay's take on death. To paraphrase:

> I think of life as a movie. We come in part way through the movie and leave before the end. The movie continues, and we move on.

PART II

PRACTICAL

Herbal first aid

Natural quick fixes: A–Z

Aches and pains

CBD patches are great for localised pain, and I use CBD Brothers (www.cbdbrothers.com).

Ointments like infused chilli oil are good for dull aches and pulled muscles.

Daisy ointment is great for bruises and knocks.

For ongoing, chronic pain, osteopathy and acupuncture will give short-term relief, but the long term only exercise and herbal medicine will fix this.

Pilates is great for the for lower back, as it works on the core muscles at the front of the body, which support the back muscles. There are plenty of online tutorials if you don't fancy being among the 'leotard ladies'. Lots of dancers practice Pilates.

Gentle yoga works well to re-educate the back and shoulders for long-term relief. The downward dog pose is especially good for lower back pain. My favourite yoga teachers are Kino, who run an online yoga school for all levels (www.omstars. com) but also has lots of free classes on YouTube. Laruga (www. larugayogacom) is more advanced but gives good beginners classes. There are loads on YouTube. David Garrigues gives a lot of philosophy in his teaching (www.davidgarrigues.com). Many yoga studios offer online classes, such as www.indabay-oga.com and www.triyoga.co.uk. Iyengar Yoga London (www. iyengaryogalondon.co.uk) offers classes for the over 60s (in person only), but there may be others in your area.

Neck pain may be caused by too much phone and laptop use or wear and tear and stress on the neck. Again, yoga stretching can help. I have found neck stretchers really useful; you can buy a variety at www.kenkoback.com

Circulation

As we age, our circulation slows, which is why we grow colder and swollen ankles and legs and varicose veins can be an issue. I have found EMS machines (electro-muscle stimulation) especially helpful; they send a gentle pulse of electricity through your legs which improves circulation and leg pain. There are several on the market, but the one I use is www.manomano.co.uk

Raising the legs will help. Walking for 30 minutes a day is especially useful to get the circulation moving.

Taking circulatory stimulants like rosemary and ginger can help, and also liver remedies as varicose veins can be caused by backflow from the liver (see Materia Medica). If they are severe or you have deep vein issues (DVT) please contact a professional herbalist for your treatment.

Witch hazel hydrosol gives relief from itchy varicose veins, while horse chestnut lotion can also give some relief.

Coughs and colds

For prevention, take fire cider, garlic honey, ginger, or elderber-ries during the winter months. Anything hot and spicy helps, like chilli and a nice cough mix can be made from onions.

Chest rubs of eucalyptus essential oil diluted in a carrier oil like almond oil or olbas oil are really helpful (5 drops to 50 ml of oil).

Cough mixtures like Liquorice and Thyme both soothe and fight the infection (see Materia Medica).

Vitamin C in large does also helps (1 g or more) as does zinc.

Avoid mucus-producing foods such as dairy, refined carbohydrates, and sugar, and eat lots of garlic, onions, and chilli-type foods.

Inhalations really help to loosen thick mucus in the lungs and calm cough. Add 5 drops of either eucalyptus or rosemary or 3 drops of tee tree or thyme essential oil.

don't take essential oils internally except under supervision

Cystitis

Drink as much filtered water as you can bear to flush out the infection. Teas of corn silk, marshmallow, comfrey leaf, and dandelion herb are helpful in large quantities. Dandelion is especially useful as it contains potassium which is lost with pharmaceutical diuretics.

For prevention, drink large quantities of water daily, a minimum of 1 litre, and avoid irritants like alcohol, tea, coffee and cigarettes.

Don't use synthetic body washes and 'hygiene products' or bath salts and oils, all of which are irritants. If you take baths, clean the bath with gentle, natural cleaners like vinegar and lemon. Synthetic cleaners can leave a residue which inflames the mucous membranes of the vagina.

Digestive issues

Certainly, our digestion becomes slower as we age. Bitter remedies such as dandelion root, and milk thistle, and aromatic digestives such as ginger, lemon, and peppermint will all help.

Antacids suppress the secretion of stomach acids, which solves the issue short term, but the long term makes the condition worse. Herbs support digestion and its secretions.

We may have to change our diet, to a simpler one as fats especially are harder to digest as we age.

Drinking lots of liquids helps constipation which may be due to dehydration. Eating bulky food full of fibre such as psyllium seeds, vegetables, apples, celery, and cabbage adds bulk waste to our system, which moves everything along.

Diarrhoea is usually a reaction to something indigestible, such as fatty food. Otherwise, is may be a food intolerance, which can develop as we age. Eat fibre-dense foods and avoid trigger foods.

Ears

Do not put anything in the ears

Rub essential oils like rosemary diluted in a carrier oil or mullein oil behind the ear for earaches. Not much can be done about deafness, but mucus-inducing foods will block the ears making the hearing worse.

Energy

Energy slumps, especially after eating or mid-afternoon, are often due to insulin resistance, avoid sugar, eat healthy meals full of protein and fibre, eat at the same time every day, have your main meal at lunchtime.

Energy balls, rosemary, and nettle seeds are stimulants and can be used as a pick-me-up (see Materia Medica).

Eyes

For mild irritation of the eyes, use chamomile (the teabags will work). Make a strong tea with half a cup of boiling water and two teabags. Allow to cool and make an eyebath from the tea and/or lay a teabag on each eye.

If the irritation is stronger or you feel there might be an infection, make a similarly strong tea of calendula and bathe the eyes-be sure not to cross-contaminate, and use a different pad for each eye.

Weleda also make nice eye drops. If you can get it, Eyebright (*Euphrasia officinalis*) is a great herbal remedy for the eyes; it grows wild in Scotland and the North.

Cornflower hydrosol is great for red, irritated eyes; I spritz it over closed eyes for instant relief (www.oshadhi.co.uk). Rose-water is also helpful and is widely available.

Traynor (www.traynor.co.uk) pinhole glasses are great for tired eyes, lots of screen watching and blurred vision.

The Bates method (www.thebatesmethod.com) has exercises you can do to improve your vision.

Nutrition: Vitamin A is helpful for the eyes, including poor vision in dim light and night vision. Good sources are cod liver oil, liver, carrots, egg yolks, cheese, butter, milk, green vegetables, yellow, and orange fruit and vegetables.

A deficiency of B2 can lead to bloodshot blurry eyes, a burning or gritty feeling in the eyes, and sensitivity to bright lights. Good food sources include yeast extract, nutritional yeast, wholegrains, and bee pollen.

Vitamin C may help in the prevention of glaucoma and cataracts. Healthy eyes contain high quantities of Vitamin C. Sources include kiwi fruit, citrus fruit, tomatoes and green vegetables.

Vitamin E is believed to prevent cataracts and keep the blood vessels and retina healthy. Sources include wholegrains, wheatgerm, and avocados.

Selenium slows the ageing of the eye. Sources include sesame and sunflower seeds, Brazil nuts, wholegrains, fish, and shellfish.

The retina needs high quantities of zinc to function properly. Zinc releases Vitamin A from the liver. Sources include egg yolks, nuts and seeds, sardines, liver, shellfish and red meat.

Eye exercises

Palming: covering your eyes with your hands revives tired eyes. As you cover your eyes look up and down and right and left, repeat ten times.

Focus on an object at arm's length, then slowly bring it close until it touches your nose. Do this slowly. Repeat ten times.

Footcare

Check your shoes: Birkenstock, Crocs, and Vivobarefoot all do shoes which are a more natural shape to help with foot pain.

Massaging your feet nightly with a nice foot oil like almond or infused comfrey or calendula oil helps to keep the skin soft and prevent cracking. Pop on a pair of socks afterwards, and you will wake up with soft feet.

Hair

Hair naturally thins as we grow older. Omega 3 capsules are helpful. I use the vegan ones form www.nothingfishy.co

Environmental toxins, poor diet and stress affect hair growth.

Herbal teas can be used as a final rinse. Nettle is a favourite or chamomile. You can massage growth-promoting oils into your scalp. A hair tonic I like is from www.laztheplantscientist.com

Hair tonic

This is best made with fresh herbs, although dried herbs can be used.

- Take one handful of rosemary leaves and flowers (discard the woody stem) and one handful of nettle leaves.
- Cut up into small pieces (2 cm) with scissors.
- Put in a large saucepan and cover with cold water so the water is around 4 cm above the herbs.
- Bring to the boil and simmer for around 30 minutes with the lid on. Leave to cool and strain.
- Pour over the hair repeatedly, and catch it in a bowl to pour again.
- Massage your scalp with your fingertips. Allow the hair to dry naturally (i.e. not with a hair drier) if possible, ideally in the sunshine. You can store any leftover in the fridge; it will last a couple of days.
- Repeat as often as you can.

Check your shampoo and conditioner are the most gentle/ natural as you can find or wash your hair with good, natural soap and then use the tonic afterwards. If your hair tends towards greasy, add a teaspoon of apple cider vinegar to the tonic. I use soaps from www.littlebirdsoaps.com, which are handmade by a herbalist, using her home grown herbs and are gentle on the skin and hair.

Headaches

My favourite headache remedies include a double expresso (increases circulation of blood to the brain), either a few drops of rosemary essential oil on the forehead and temples (dull headaches) or lavender (stress related), a long walk in the fresh air, strong ginger tea, a shot of fire cider, the juice of a lemon diluted in water, and peppermint tea.

Headaches are symptoms. They are the body's way of calling our attention to an imbalance. We may have headaches due to liver congestion (one-sided, at the temples), or at the base of the skull (tension), or around the face (nerve pain from teeth or blocked sinuses). Viruses give dull headaches, which can be resistant to treatment, except fire cider, which I have found helps as it deals with the virus rather than the headache.

Drops of lavender essential oil in a bath may help tension headaches, as will linden blossom tea. For knock out to sleep it off, use wild lettuce glycerite.

If you do yoga, a headstand will often do the trick (although it feels rather strange), followed by a shoulder stand.

Skin

The skin is the largest organ of the body. What we put on our skin is absorbed into the bloodstream. Be careful, then, if you have skin issues, of what chemicals come in contact with your skin. From washing powders, shower gels, shampoos, conditioners, skin creams, body lotions, cleaning chemicals, etc., organic is best; www.peacewiththewild.co.uk sells nice products. You can make your own household cleansers (Clean and Green by Nancy Birtwhistle has some nice recipes). (See Materia Medica for recipes for skin cream.)

Sleep

Knock-out remedies include chamomile (mild), lavender (medium), wild lettuce, and hops (strong) (see Rest for more ideas).

Teeth and gums

Oil pulling has been shown to help with bad breath, inflamed gums, and gingivitis. This involves taking a teaspoon to a tablespoon of coconut oil and swilling it around your mouth for 5–20 minutes, and then spitting it out (don't spit it down the sink as it will harden and cause a blockage). The oil draws out pathogens from the gums and teeth. Brush your teeth well afterwards. Do 4–7 times a week. (see Materia Medica for other oil-pulling mixtures.)

For local inflammation and pain, rub calendula tincture over the affected area.

Use a natural toothpaste and mouthwashes (see Materia Medica). Antiseptic herbs like calendula and thyme can be made into mouthwashes (use a strong tea and swill around the mouth for 5–10 minutes).

Liquorice tincture helps rebuild gum tissue. Frankincense also rebuilds the gums. Yarrow and tee tree are anti-inflammatory (see Materia Medica).

Viruses

We are susceptible to viruses when our immunity is low. For prevention, take fire cider or elderberry syrup during the winter months.

If you start to feel ill, then up your dose of fire cider or elderberry, take raw garlic, or onion and drink lots of water. High doses of Vitamin C are helpful too: 1–2 g every hour until symptoms subside.

Your medicine cabinet

In your pantry

There are many remedies that are normal cooking ingredients which we can use to promote health and wellbeing.

- Chilli.
- Garlic.
- Ginger.
- Horseradish.

- Lemons.
- Onions.
- Turmeric.

In your garden and wildcrafting

These herbal remedies are easy to grow in pots or can be picked in the wild (see section on wildcrafting herbs).

- Agrimony.
- Borage.
- Calendula.
- Chamomile.
- Dandelion.
- Elderflowers and berries.
- Hawthorn flowers berries.
- Hops.
- Lavender.
- Lemon balm.
- Linden blossom.
- Mushrooms.
- Rosemary.
- Sage.
- Thyme.
- Yarrow.

Buy-ins

These are best bought from a reliable supplier. Choose one that specialises in herbs, so they are fresh.

- Milky oats (these can also be found wild).
- Horse chestnut.
- Milk thistle.

- Skullcap.
- Passiflora.
- Witch hazel.
- Liquorice.

Herbal first aid kit

- Marigold tincture.
- Daisy balm.
- CBD patches.
- Lavender essential oil.
- Rosemary essential oil.
- Eucalyptus essential oil.
- Marigold cream.
- Rosewater hydrosol.
- Fire cider.
- Liquorice and thyme cough mix.
- Washable cotton make up pads.

Making herbal remedies

If you can cook, you can easily make your own remedies; no special equipment is required, just saucepans, jars, bottles, and bowls plus a hand mixture or electric mixer.

Herbal tea

Herbal teas are taken in much stronger doses than herbal tea bags, which are available to buy. There is really no comparison if you are looking for herbal healing. I recommend you buy organic herbs wherever possible or wildcraft the herbs if you are able to. If you can get a special jug or teapot, this is ideal. Try to make a ritual of taking your herbal tea, as self-care is part of any healing process. If you can, brew your tea and take a moment to sit and drink it slowly and mindfully, visualising the healing benefits flooding your cells. Of the suggested mixture, take 1 tablespoon full (15 g) and pour on 250–300 ml of boiling water (depending on the type of herb, roots require less water, very leafy herbs a bit more). Cover and allow to sit for 10–15 minutes. Strain and drink unsweetened. If the taste is a bit strong, then dilute it with water to make it palatable.

Suppliers

www.caleysapothecary.co.uk/ – all organic produce is sourced by a trained medical herbalist.

www.baldwins.co.uk – sell both organic and non-organic herbs. They also sell nice glass teapots.

There may be a herbal apothecary near you. Check the herbs are not stored in the window (sunlight degrades them), and they have a fairly brisk turnover (so the herbs are not old).

If you wish to learn to forage your own herbs or grow them, check out herbalists on Instagram, many of whom do herb walks in the summer months. The Herb Society has details of herb growers at https://herbsociety.org.uk

Herbal baths

Herbal baths are like lying in a warm herbal infusion.

- Take a muslin cloth,[141] or a large handkerchief and put a handful of the herbs inside.
- Tie tightly under the hot tap, allowing the hot water to slowly run through.
- Alternatively, run the bath and put the herb into the bath and allow it to steep for 5–10 minutes in the hot water (like a teabag in hot water).

- Then add cold water to suit and sit in the bath for as long as feels comfortable.
- Do be sure the bath has not been cleaned with harsh chemicals as you don't want to absorb these.

Hand and foot baths

These work very well if you don't want to lie in a bath.

- Make a strong tea and pour it into some warm water.
- Immerse your hands of feet in the water for 10–15 minutes until the water grows cold.
- Fresh herbs are good for hand and foot baths. You can use, melissa, lavender, calendula, comfrey herb, and drop 5 drops of essential oil in the bath.

Tinctures

Tinctures are alcoholic extracts of herbs; they allow us to collect herbs at their peak and preserve their active ingredients for later use. Tinctures, because they are made from alcohol, last indefinitely.

I make my tinctures with vodka, which is the purest alcohol. Always dry the herb before making the tinctures to reduce the water content.

- In a large glass jar, fill with the dried herb until the jar is almost full.
- Pour on the vodka, press down until the herb is covered and there are 5 cm of liquid above the herb.
- Stand in a dark place for four weeks, shaking the jar occasionally to make sure all the herb is covered.
- Strain through a muslin cloth or fine sieve.
- Label and bottle.
- Dose 10 drops three times daily.[142]

Infused oils — slow and fast methods.

These are not essential oils, which are made using an alembic.

- Pick your herb and allow it to wilt for a couple of days to reduce the water content.
- Place in a clean glass jar leaving a little space at the top.
- Fill the jar with a good oil, either organic olive oil, almond oil or Hempseed oil.
- Push the herb down so it is completely covered by the oil.
- Stand in a sunny windowsill for a few weeks; the oil will change colour.
- Check the herb is completely submerged from time to time.

Clearly, this works only in summer. At other times you can slowly heat the herb and oil mixture in a *bain marie*, taking care not to overheat the oil. I heat it up until the water underneath is boiling, then turn the heat off and repeat several times over the course of a few days. You can also do this is a slow cooker. Turn it on and off over the course of a few days.

Herbs to make oils from include: calendula, comfrey, lavender, chilli, rosemary, lemon balm, and yarrow.

Store in a cool, dark place or in the fridge.

Herbal balms and creams

The herbal oil is the basis for balms and creams.

Balms

In a *bain marie* heat 100 ml of infused oil …

- Add 1 teaspoon of beeswax (add more or less depending on how solid you want your balm).
- Add 1 tablespoon of coconut oil.
- Add 4–6 drops of essential oil.

- Gently warm and dissolve the first three ingredients.
- Remove from the heat and beat with a hand mixture until it cools and solidifies.
- Drop the essential oils in and beat again.
- Pour into glass jars and keep in the fridge.
- Add lavender essential oil for cooling and pain relieving, tee tree or thyme for antiseptic action, and plantain infused oil for insect bites.

Creams

- Add 100 ml rosewater or other flower waters like orange blossom, elderflower, and rose geranium.
- Add 25 ml of almond oil or any other nice oil such as jojoba, avocado, or argan oil.
- Add 25 g mango butter or other butter like coconut butter, Shea butter, avocado butter etc.
- Heat the rosewater and the oil and butter in two *bain maries* until they are at a similar temperature, if you have a thermometer, around 70 degrees Celsius.
- Mix both liquids together, beating until they cool and become fluffy.
- Pot up and keep in the fridge.
- You can add 5 drops of essential oil if you wish once the mixture has thickened. Rose geranium or vanilla are nice smelling for skincare.

Using essential oils

Essential oils are very strong concentrations of herbs. They can be added in small quantities to baths and creams. If you are applying them to the skin, always dilute them with a carrier oil like almond oil. They may burn otherwise. Do not go into strong sunlight if you have essential oils on your skin. They may burn or cause a rash. Please use them sparingly.

Do not take essential oils internally

Using essential oils

Don't take essential oils internally; they are very strong and can be toxic in this form.

- Use a good carrier oil: I like almond oil, but jojoba, avocado, and any other good quality oil will do. If possible, use organic oils, both carrier oil and essential oil.
- Pour some oil into the palm of your hand and drop 5 drops of the essential oil into the oil.
- Rub your palms together to heat up and mix the two oils.
- Apply as indicated and cover with a cotton cloth or tee shirt until the oil has been absorbed.

Good quality oils will absorb the quickest.

For inhalation, take a mixing bowl full of boiling water and drop 5 drops of the oil into the water. Cover your head with a towel and breathe in the steam as deeply as you are able to.

If you are applying to the lungs, rub the oil over the front, sides, and back from the neck to the bottom of the rib cage (as far as you can reach) and cover with a cotton tee shirt.

Essential oils can also be dropped into bathwater (unless you have skin issues). Drop 5 drops into the bath water once drawn and lie in the warm water for as long as you can. Soap and shower gel will disperse the oil, so use these baths as a treatment and not for washing.

Of course, not all bodies are the same. If the dose is too high, cut down the essential oil to 2 or 3 drops or increase up to 7 drops if it feels too low. Always dilute with a carrier oil and use 1–2 times daily maximum. If you have skin issues, start with the lowest dose and patch test an area to determine your tolerance. If in doubt, stop using it or use it as an inhalation instead.

Using hydrosols

Hydrosols, also called hydrolats, and flower waters, are aromatic herbs extracted by using a still or alembic. After the essential oil has been distilled, the floral waters are made. Common hydrosols are rose water, orange blossom, and rose geranium. They can be taken internally and spritzed on the body. Rosewater is great for hot, irritated skin; orange blossom and lavender are cooling and calming remedies. The actions of the hydrosols are the same as the herb as a tea or tincture.

Vinegars

Another way to extract and preserve herbs is to infuse them in vinegar, always use the best cider vinegar you can find. I infuse citrus fruit rinds in vinegar which works as a lovely digestive. Only use unwaxed or organic fruit for this.

- Fill a large glass jar with the vinegar and add the roughly chopped rind, making sure they are covered with the liquid. Leave for around a month, and then strain and bottle.
- You may wish to add honey to the vinegar (which makes an oxymel) to take them, gently warm the strained vinegar, remove from the heat, and stir in honey or coconut sugar to taste.
- Take a shot-glass full or dilute in a glass of water daily, especially with slow digestion, constipation and wind or nausea.

Glycerites

For people who don't want to use alcoholic tinctures, glycerites offer an alternative.

Melissa, cleavers, and wild lettuce make great glycerites.

Use vegetable glycerine. You can make glycerites from fresh herbs, which is another advantage.

- Pick your fresh herb, chop or mash it into a pulp and cover it with the glycerine leaving around 3 cm of liquid above the herb.
- Leave for a couple of weeks, pressing down the herb to make sure it is covered and then strain and bottle.
- I store glycerites in the fridge as they don't last as well as tinctures.
- The dose is a tablespoon full, as required.

Detox tea blend

- Cleavers.
- Dandelion herb.
- Elderflower.
- Marigold.

Calm tea

- Rose petals.
- Melissa.
- Chamomile.
- Oat straw.

Sleepy tea

- Lime flowers.
- Melissa.
- ½ quantity of hop flowers.
- Elderflowers.

Immune tea

- Marigold flowers.
- Cleavers.

- Nettle.
- Yarrow.
- Thyme.

Healthy heart tea

Equal parts of …

- Hawthorn berries.
- Linden blossom.
- Pinch of ginger.
- Rosemary.
- Rose buds.

Happy gut tea

- Equal parts of dried.
- Fennel.
- Dandelion root.
- Agrimony.
- Lemon or orange peel.
- Rosemary.

Hop pillow

Mix 75 g each of dried …

- Lavender flowers.
- Rosebuds.
- Hop flowers.
- Linden Blossom in a cotton bag.

Cover the bag with a pillowcase (so it can be washed).

Stress-busting tea

- Hawthorn blossoms.
- Melissa.

- Linden blossom.
- Rose buds.

Cystitis tea

Mix equal parts …

- Corn silk.
- Horsetail.
- Dandelion herb.
- Marshmallow root.
- ½ amount of thyme.

Elderberry syrup

- 500 g elderberries (no stalks or leaves).
- 5 star anise flowers.
- 2 cinnamon quills.
- 1 litre of cold water.
- Bring to the boil and simmer until the liquid is reduced to 300 ml.
- Strain and add 300 g of sugar (cane, muscovado, coconut).
- Heat very gently to dissolve sugar, stirring constantly.
- Remove from heat and allow to cool completely.
- Bottle and label and keep in the fridge.
- Take 1 tablespoon daily neat or in a little water.
- The proportions for syrups are 1 part liquid to 1 part sugar.

Other herbs you can make syrups from include rose petals, melissa, and any of the cough remedies.

Garlic honey

- In a new jar of honey, pour out the top 20% of the honey.
- Peel and chop the cloves from a whole bulb of garlic (organic if possible).

- Add to jar and stir well.
- Top up the jar with the remaining honey until the jar is full.
- Leave for 2–3 weeks.
- Take 1–2 teaspoons daily as a preventative.
- For cough, take a teaspoon every couple of hours neat or in warm water.

If this is too strong, then you can use onions instead of garlic

Slice the onions thinly. In a large glass jar, put a layer of onions, they a layer of honey or sugar, then another layer of onions, then sugar. Repeat until all the onions have been used. Finish with a thick layer of sugar or honey. Leave for 2–3 weeks. Take a teaspoon every couple of hours neat or in water.

Rose honey

This is a beautiful remedy for sadness, and shock, and whenever you need comfort, use fresh rose petals, and make sure they have not been sprayed.

Other kinds of honey include melissa honey, rosemary honey, and lavender honey.

- Pack the jar as described for onion honey, pressing down each layer.
- Leave for 3–4 weeks and take as above.

Liquorice and thyme cough mixture

- 50 g of liquorice root.
- A handful of fresh thyme or 1 dessertspoon of dried.
- 1 litre of cold water.

- 250 g coconut or unrefined sugar.
- Put the root in the water in a strong saucepan. Bring to the boil slowly and simmer with the lid on for 20 minutes. Allow to cool. Then bring to the boil again and simmer. Repeat 4–5 times, leaving overnight if possible.
- Bring to the boil and simmer to reduce to 300 ml.
- Add the Thyme and simmer for another 30 minutes covered.
- Strain into a measuring jug. It needs to be 250 ml; if less, add water; if too much, simmer and reduce.
- Add the strained liquid to the cleaned pan and add 250 g of coconut sugar or other sugar and over a low heat, dissolve the sugar completely, stirring all the time.
- Allow to cool and bottle in sterilised bottles.
- Dose: 1–2 teaspoons 3–4 times a day.

You could also use the following:

- Elecampane root.
- White horehound herb.
- Mullein.

Iron tonic

Because our digestion gets less efficient, we can suffer from anaemia as we grow older. Vegetarians and vegans especially need to be aware of their iron consumption. This tonic is easy to make and pleasant tasting and has the benefit of not causing constipation which pharmaceutical iron can do.

- 20 g dried nettle leaves.
- 30 g yellow dock root.
- 20 g horsetail.
- 20 g dandelion root.
- The peel and juice of one organic lemon.
- 40 g hunza apricots chopped.

- In a large saucepan, mix all the ingredients, and cover with spring water, pushing the herbs down to make sure they are covered by the liquid. Bring to the boil and simmer for 15 minutes. Turn off the heat. Repeat several times over the next two days.
- After the last heating, strain and add 2 tablespoons of molasses to the liquid, stir until it has dissolved.
- Dose: 1 tablespoon as required.

Wine method – red wine contains iron and is useful to make the iron tonic, and of course, it tastes fabulous!

- Cover the ingredients in a large, glass jar with organic red wine.
- Leave for a few weeks, strain and over a low heat add 3 tablespoonfuls of molasses, stirring until it has dissolved. The heat will burn off the alcohol.
- Dose: a teaspoonful daily neat or in warm water.
- Keep refrigerated.

You can substitute apple cider vinegar for the wine if you wish.

Fire cider

The ingredients can vary according to what is in season; generally, hot and spicy foods need to be added, plus a citrus fruit and a few herbs. Try to use organic ingredients.

- In a large jar, add …
- 1 garlic bulb chopped.
- 3 inches (7.5 cm) of fresh ginger root grated.
- 2–3 red chillies chopped.
- 1 lemon chopped.
- A handful of nettle leaves.
- A handful of rosemary.

- A handful of thyme chopped.
- Cover with cider vinegar (organic and with the mother if possible), so there are about 4 cm of liquid above the ingredients.
- Cover with a lid or a muslin cloth.
- Shake the jar so that everything is well mixed, pushing the ingredients down under the liquid.
- Leave in a dark place for a month shaking every day.
- Strain the liquid and gently warm it in a saucepan.
- Stir in honey or coconut sugar to taste; it is strong, so it does need a sweetener.
- Dose: take a tablespoonful in water daily during the flu season.

You can also use horseradish, onion (if garlic is too fiery), stronger chilli like Scotch Bonnet, and turmeric (you will have to add black pepper and a spoonful of coconut oil to extract it properly).

Fire cider is also a great digestive remedy; all that heat gets things moving.

if you have inflammation in your stomach or digestive tract, make a milder version and drink diluted in a large glass of water after meals

Elderflower champagne

There are so many recipes for this. I like this one as it's simple and does not make gallons of the champagne.[143]

- 1.5 litres of boiled water.
- 150 g golden sugar granulated or caster sugar.
- 1 lemon.
- 1 tablespoon cider vinegar.

- 4 fresh elderflower heads unwashed, as they have pollen on them, which acts like yeast.
- In a glass bowl, mix the boiling water and the sugar until it has dissolved, and leave to cool.
- Halve the lemon and squeeze the juice. Add juice and lemon skin to the bowl.
- Add the vinegar and stir well.
- Add the elderflower heads with the stalks removed (a fork does this well).
- Cover with a cloth and leave for 24 hours.
- Sieve the liquid and fill sterilised bottles leaving 3–4 cm at the top for gas.
- Leave for three weeks, opening the bottles every couple of days to 'burp' them and remove any gas build-up (otherwise, the bottles may explode).

Toothpaste (thanks to Dawn Ireland Herbalist for this recipe)

- 150 g kaolin (soap kitchen).
- 150 g chalk (aromantic, BP grade).
- 100 g vegetable glycerine (soap kitchen).
- 90 g liquorice tincture (any herb supplier) this has research showing plaque inhibition.
- 25 g myrrh tincture (any herb supplier) gum hardening and antiseptic.
- 20 drops essential oil of choice. I like myrrh and yarrow, but you can also use tee tree (for infections), Frankincense to harden the gums, sage for bleeding, etc.

Mouthwash

- 350 ml of liquid, you can use a variety of hydrosols. I like yarrow, sage, or a mixture.
- To 350 ml of liquid, add a mixture of essential oils.

- 10 drops Frankincense (rebuilds gum tissue, stimulates repair, anti-inflammatory).
- 5 drops of Clove essential oil (painkilling for sore gums).
- 10 drops of peppermint (refreshes the mouth).
- 5 drops of Sage essential oil (astringent for the gums).
- 2 drops tee tree (antibacterial).
- Mix everything together in a glass jar.
- Take 1 tablespoon and rinse the mouth, and then spit out.

Oil pulling recipe

You can just use coconut oil (organic if possible).

Take 1 teaspoon of oil and put it in your mouth; it will quickly melt. Swish it around your mouth for 10–20 minutes. Spit out into the bin (not down the sink, as it will block it). Brush your teeth afterwards or use a mouthwash. Do 5–7 times a week.

Sesame oil mix

- 200 ml of organic sesame oil.
- 10 drops of yarrow essential oil.
- 10 drops of frankincense essential oil.
- 5 drops of clove essential oil.
- 1–3 drops of tee tree oil.
- Mix well in a glass bottle.
- Take 2 teaspoons and swill around the mouth as described above.

You can change the essential oils as you wish.

Suncream

This cream is for just wandering about in bright sunshine. It will not work if you lie in the midday sun for hours!

Zinc reflects the sunlight away from the skin. It has a white appearance, but this soon disappears.

- 110 ml oil (jojoba, almond, avocado, etc.).
- 55 ml coconut oil.
- 30 g beeswax (use less if you want it runny).
- 1 teaspoon red raspberry seed oil (optional).
- 2 tablespoons shea butter.
- Put all the ingredients in a *bain marie*. This can be a strong jam jar in boiling water or a glass bowl.
- Melt over a low heat.
- Remove from the heat and beat with a whisk or food mixer until thick and creamy.
- Add 2 tablespoons non-nano zinc oxide (be sure to mask up or cover your nose and mouth while you do this).
- Stir until it is all mixed in.
- In strong sunshine, reapply every hour or after swimming.

Face cream

There are many complicated recipes out there; this is a simple one I use myself. Keep it in the fridge as it does not contain preservatives. It is a bit greasy at first but soon is absorbed by the skin.

- 50 g Shea butter (or mango butter or any other nice butter).
- 30 g Coconut oil.
- 50 g oil (jojoba, almond, avocado, etc.).
- 50–100 ml hydrosol (chamomile, rose, orange blossom, frankincense, etc.).
- 20 g beeswax (or less if you want more liquid).
- In a *bain marie*, slowly melt all the ingredients except the hydrosol.
- Remove from the heat and beat until thick and creamy.
- Beat in the hydrosol.
- Store in the fridge.

Hand cream

Use the above recipe. For a harder cream, add more beeswax; for a lotion, add less.

You may add a few drops of essential oil to perfume it.

Lotion

See above.

Energy balls

These are great for afternoon energy slumps and when out walking or exercising. Good quality dates can be bought from charities supporting impoverished people (https:// thedateproject.org/date-tins/).

You can change the ingredients for different kinds of nuts, peanuts, and other nut butters and ground almonds. You will need a food processor.

- 14 dates.
- +/− 200 g of mixed nuts.
- Or 100 g of nuts and 2 tablespoons of nut butter.
- Put all the ingredients in a food processor until mixed and mashed up completely.
- Form into small golf-ball-sized pieces, and roll in coconut, cocoa, cacao, or chocolate as required.
- They last around three weeks stored in the fridge.

You can also add, nettle seeds for a big energy boost, matcha powder, and moringa seeds. The combinations are endless.

Wildcrafting: etiquette and considerations

If you plan to pick your own remedies (especially mushrooms), go on a herb walk with a herbalist or forager who will show you how to identify your herbs (see Action). Pick only where the plant is growing abundantly, as this shows the soil conditions are ideal for growth. Observe the pee line. Pick plants that grow 3 foot from a path or road and 3 foot high above the path to avoid dog pee. Don't take all the plants; leave some to propagate for next year. Don't uproot herbs, except for dandelion, nettle and burdock, which are common. Don't wash the herbs or dry them in the kitchen. A dry, well-ventilated space is ideal. Hang them flowers facing downwards, or on paper, turning frequently, do not dry and store them in direct sunlight. Store in brown paper bags or jars in a cupboard. Label everything!

If you are not sure about what you are picking, go on a herb walk with a herbalist. In the spring, summer, and autumn months, herbalists lead walks in their local area. See resources for a list of herbal organisations.

Materia Medica

Agrimony (Agrimonia officinalis)

Agrimony grows wild in the UK. It is found near water, usually rivers and streams. It is an easy plant to overlook; it has small, yellow flowers, and a spindly stem. Agrimony flowers during the summer months, June, July, and August.

Part used: the flowering parts are used, the stem, leaves, and flowers. Agrimony can be taken as a tea or as a tincture.

Actions: agrimony is a great remedy for the gut. It stimulates digestion and soothes and heals the digestive tract. It is a great liver remedy where the stomach is delicate and cannot tolerate stronger bitters like milk thistle.

It is a great remedy to take alongside pharmaceuticals to help the body deal with the chemical fallout.

Use Agrimony for any post-viral lethargy and weakness, following shingles and other viral conditions, such a hepatitis and glandular fever.

Borage (Borago officinalis)

Borage grows easily and abundantly in gardens. It flowers through late spring and throughout the summer.

Part used: the flowers and leaves are used in teas and tinctures. Borage can also be used in cooking. It's a bit like spinach.

Actions: borage is an ideal herb to take when recovering from prolonged stress, trauma, viral infections, surgery, and chemotherapy. It gently nourishes and strengthens the adrenal glands (that fight-or-flight mechanism) when they have become exhausted. Borage builds up stamina slowly and safely. Use after flu to build up your strength. It is soothing to the gut and lungs and bladder, and so borage is a helpful remedy for cough, bronchitis, colds, and sore throats, for upset stomach and gastritis and cystitis.

Calendula (Calendula officinalis)

Marigold is easily cultivated in the garden. It flowers during the summer months.

Part used: we use the flowers of marigold. Marigold is taken externally as an infused oil or cream, and internally as a tea or tincture, lotion, eye bath and powder.

Actions: marigold is one of the main first aid remedies. Keep it in the form of an ointment or cream or infused oil for cuts, burns, rashes, or infected wounds, as an eyebath (the tea) for red, sore eyes, conjunctivitis, for spots, pimples, boils, and all skin irritation.

Internally, taken as a tea or tincture, marigold is a great liver remedy to promote digestion, for lack of appetite, poor digestion, bloating, and constipation. Marigold is a powerful healing remedy and can be taken to heal the digestive tract in irritable bowel syndrome, colitis gastritis and any inflammation of the gut, including mouth ulcers (use the tea as a mouthwash), gingivitis, and bleeding gums.

Marigold supports the lymphatic system, so used to promote immunity, following viral infections, tonsilitis, chronic sore throats and any conditions where the immune system is compromised.

Calendula is anti-fungal; the powder is used locally for athlete's foot, and the tincture is used for fungal nail infections both locally and internally.

Marigold makes an excellent lotion for painful varicose veins, and taken internally it will relieve liver congestion, which is often a cause of swollen veins.

As a cream, it is a standard in first aid kits as it heals wounds, especially those which are infected, also for styes and conjunctivitis and other irritating eye conditions. The tincture is useful for spots dropped directly on the spot to dry it out. Calendula can also be used for herpes sores.

CBD (Cannabis sativa/indica)

I get mine from CBD Brothers (www.cbdbrothers.com). I especially like their CBD patches which you can apply for localised pain.

It is illegal to grow cannabis. The penalty is up to 14 years in prison.

Chamomile (Anthemis nobilis)

Chamomile is easily cultivated in the garden or window box. It flowers during the summer months.

Part used: we use the flowers and leaves of chamomile as a tea, essential oil, hydrosol, ointment, tincture, and lotion.

Actions: Chamomile is a gentle, soothing remedy for the gut and nervous system. Any digestive problems caused by anxiety or stress like diarrhoea, constipation, acid reflux, stomach pains, IBS, and gastritis.

Chamomile has a gentle bitterness, and so it stimulates the appetite and increases the digestion and absorption of food.

Chamomile is relaxing and comforting to the nervous system, use for headaches, palpitations, tension, anxiety, mild insomnia, and interrupted sleep.

Chamomile is a great tea to drink in the evenings to prepare for sleeping. The essential oil of chamomile can be added to a warm bath before bed (3–5 drops) or sprinkled on the pillow for a restful sleep.

Chamomile is a great soothing, pain-relieving remedy for mouth and gum issues to relieve and heal inflammation and irritation there. Use the hydrosol or a strong tea as a mouthwash, use the tincture locally for sore spots in the mouth.

Chamomile is a great remedy for the skin. The hydrosol is used as a toner and will dry up spots and cool rashes.

Chilli (Capsicum spp.)

Chillies can be grown in the garden and greenhouse.

Part used: green and red chillies are used as remedies. If you are buying them in, try to buy organic chillies. Chillies are used as infused oils, in cooking and in fire cider.

Actions: chillies are super-hot, and so kill viruses, bacteria, and other pathogens by raising the body's temperature (fever works in this way). They are helpful as an infused oil for muscle pain but do a skin-patch test first as not all skin types tolerate this much heat.

Besides local treatment, chillies are an ingredient of fire cider which is a preventative remedy taken in the winter months against viral infections, colds, and flu.

Fire cider is also a great remedy for poor digestion, bloating and gas, as it heats the stomach and gets digestion going.

Avoid where there is inflammation, such as stomach ulcers, gastritis, colitis, IBS, etc.

Chilli oil can be used (in small quantities) with other lung remedies such as a chest rub to get cold, damp phlegm out of the body.

Dandelion *(*Taraxacum officinalis*)*

Dandelions grow everywhere! Dig up the root in early spring before the flowers appear and in late autumn when the leaves are falling. Leaves and flowers can be picked between those times.

Part used: the flowering parts, flowers, and leaves are used for the lungs and kidneys. The root is used for the liver. Both are taken as tea, powder, and tincture.

Actions: as one of the first plants that grow in spring, dandelion is used as a spring green cooked or raw in salads.

Root

The root contains bitters, and so is a liver remedy. As a bitter, it should be taken 20 minutes before food and swilled around the mouth, so the taste buds get the full sensation of bitterness. Dandelion is a great all-round liver healing remedy, so used in liver conditions such as poor digestion, bloating, and acid reflux.

Dandelion is especially helpful in constipation as it doesn't work by irritating the bowel (like Senna) but instead increases digestive enzymes, which invigorate the whole digestive tract, getting things moving.

Dandelion cleanses the blood as so is used in inflammatory conditions such as arthritis, eczema, urticaria, psoriasis and gout (with support from a herbalist). Use during chemotherapy and other drug therapies to support liver function.

The liver is often congested in varicose veins due to constipation and a sedentary lifestyle. This causes a backflow to the leg veins leading to swollen veins and haemorrhoids. Internal use of the tea or tincture will ease congestion of the liver and so relieve the symptoms.

Dandelion root is helpful in regulating high and low blood sugar, and so is a very useful remedy to take when changing your diet to reduce insulin resistance (see Nourishment). Dandelion root is one of the herbs you can take long-term.

Herb

Dandelion herbs (or greens) work on the lungs and kidneys.

Dandelion is a strong diuretic (hence its French name, *pis en lit*), but it has the benefit of containing potassium, chemical diuretics leach potassium from the body, and this is why potassium is often prescribed with them. Diuretics are used to lower high blood pressure (by reducing fluid in the body). However, if you have low blood pressure (hypotension), avoid dandelion. Dandelion soothes the bladder and can be helpful with other remedies for cystitis and urethritis (thyme).

Dandelion is used with other remedies (such as coltsfoot) for the lungs in cases of chronic cough, asthma, and bronchitis to strengthen lung tissue.

Fasting and spring cleanse. Dandelion is a great remedy to take during a fast or cleanse to get the organs of elimination going: the lungs, kidneys, and liver, to flush out the system.

Elderflower (Sambucus nigra)

Elderflowers blossom in May and June (depending on what time spring appears).

Part used: we use the flowers only. Use as a tea, hydrosol, lotion, tincture, syrup, and, of course, elderflower champagne!

Actions: elderflower is a wonderful remedy for spring colds and flu, taken as a tea or tincture. The tea tastes delicious! Elderflower releases stuck phlegm in the head in sinusitis, colds, and catarrh. Excess mucus can be an inflammatory response (see Nourishment), especially to sugar, refined carbohydrates, and dairy products, so do check your diet as well.

Elderflower increases sweating, and to reduce a fever (diaphoretic), taken hot as a tea, it can help to sweat out colds and flu.

Elderflower hydrosol or tea is used to brighten the skin and clear the complexion, as a toner and is soothing for skin rashes and irritation.

Elderflower has a gentle sedative effect and is helpful for mild insomnia, restless sleep and nightmares, tension headaches, anxiety, and stress.

Elderflower regulates the fluid balance in the body and so is helpful for water retention, sluggishness, and lethargy.

Elderberries (Sambucus nigra)

Elderberries are collected in late summer and early autumn.

Part used: the berries only (try using the prongs of a fork to separate them from the stems). Elderberries are taken as a syrup or as a tincture.

Actions: elderberries have a stronger anti-viral action than the flowers, and so are used in a similar way to fire cider, as a protective remedy against winter colds and flu. They work well mixed with ginger, cloves, and cinnamon.

Garlic (Alium sativum)

Garlic grows easily in pots and gardens. Harvest in late summer.

Part used: the fresh cloves peeled and chopped, use in garlic honey and fire cider.

Actions: garlic is used to heat and dry the body. It is an irritant, so do not use it where there is inflammation, such as stomach ulcers, sensitive, inflamed skin, etc. Garlic is anti-fungal, anti-viral, and is excreted through the lungs (hence the smell on the breath). Garlic, taken raw, finely chopped, and washed down with a glass of water, is an excellent remedy at the beginning of a cold or flu. Garlic in fire cider and garlic honey as a preventative remedy for colds and flu.

Garlic has been shown to have a beneficial effect on the heart and circulation, and eating garlic on a daily basis has been shown to reduce cholesterol levels (probably due to its anti-inflammatory action).[145]

Cooking with garlic is an ideal way to take garlic on a daily basis. After peeling and chopping the garlic, leave to sit for around ten minutes to allow the sulphur compounds (allicin) to form before adding to your cooking.

Ginger (Zingiberis officinalis)

Ginger can be grown in pots or in the garden.

Part used: the fresh, peeled, grated root in ginger syrup, in elderberry syrup, in fire cider, as an essential oil and tincture.

Actions: ginger is warming and drying, but less so than garlic, so it can be used with delicate stomachs. Ginger is an excellent remedy to take during the winter months as it prevents colds and flu and warms up the body, expelling phlegm. Add 3–5 drops of the essential oil of ginger to a steam inhalation for catarrh, sinus problems, and cough. Add the same amount to a foot bath or a regular bath to heat up a chilled body (do not use it if you have inflammatory skin conditions).

Ginger is warming, and so adding it to your daily diet stimulates digestion and can be helpful for painful joints and poor circulation in the hands and feet.

Ginger is an anti-spasmodic and digestive remedy for bloating, reflux, and sluggish digestion. Take a small piece (1 inch/2.5 cm) in warm water in the mornings to get your digestion going.

Ginger is used for nausea and dizziness, to bring blood to the head, and to treat low blood pressure.

Hawthorn blossom (Crataegus spp.)

These are picked in May usually and are widespread throughout the country.

Part used: the flowers only. Fresh or dried. Hawthorn blossom can be used as a tea, a hydrosol, or a tincture.

Actions: the flowers have a sedative action on the nerves and help to lower blood pressure due to stress (the tea is best here). Hawthorn increases peripheral circulation and so is useful for cold hands and feet and bad circulation. Useful for insomnia and a stress-busting tea (see above). The hydrosol is used to calm and relax, and it also softens the skin and makes a gentle toner.

Hawthorn berries (Crataegus spp.)

Like the flowers, these can be foraged. They are widespread and usually ripe around September or October time.

Part used: the dried berries in tea and tincture, and Healthy Heart Tea. Hawthorn berries also make a great ketchup.

Actions: Hawthorn berries are one of the main remedies herbalists use for high blood pressure, heart disease, and circulation issues (best undertaken under supervision).

The berries are healing to the arteries, the heart muscles, the capillaries, and the circulation in the brain. They reduce swelling due to heart conditions.

Hops *(Humulus lupulus)*

Hops can be grown or found growing wild in the southern parts of the country.

Part used: the strobiles (flowers) in tincture, hop pillow in hand and foot baths and as a poultice for local pain.

Actions: hops are very bitter and so are a great remedy to stimulate digestion and reduce bloating, constipation, and lethargy. They are laxatives without irritating.

They are a powerful relaxant, so do not take them before operating heavy machinery or driving. They can be taken for insomnia, one hour before retiring, headaches and migraine during an attack and long-term for strong anxiety and conditions caused by stress such a peptic ulcers, IBS, etc.

Hops can be used to dull the pain of earache, toothache, and itchy skin conditions such as shingles, ringworm. They bring boils and abscesses to a head if made into a warm poultice.

Hops may aggravate severe depression, so avoid them in this case.

Horse chestnut *(Aesculus hippocastanum.)*

Horse chestnut trees are found in parks and gardens and growing wild.

Part used: use the early leaves in spring and the conkers in autumn; use as a lotion.

Actions: horse chestnut is a strong astringent and is used to alleviate the pains in varicose veins. Make a lotion of the early leaves.

Conkers contain saponins (from which soap came) which make an alternative form of washing liquid.

Horseradish

Horseradish can be grown and found in good greengrocers.

Part used: the root, grated in food, is used in a fire cider or as a warming foot bath after a chill. It is very fiery, don't take it if you have a sensitive stomach or heat or redness or inflammation. You can get horseradish powder and tincture.

Actions: horseradish is hot and dry, more than ginger and garlic, less than chillies. Use sparingly to heat and dry the body internally. Horseradish can be used externally for pain, grated, and wrapped in a handkerchief or piece of cloth. Being spicy, it dries up mucus, and the fresh gated root in cider vinegar can help to expel the accumulation of phlegm (1/2–2 teaspoons in a cup of vinegar). Sip during the day. It is digestive and helps sluggish digestion or after a heavy meal.

Lavender (Lavendula officinalis)

Lavender is easily grown in the summer months.

Part used: the flowers are used, generally dried, and added to tea, or used as an essential oil, as a hydrosol, lotion, or tincture.

Actions: lavender is calming to the nervous system, and so a gentle tea (lavender is strong tasting, so use sparingly) or foot or hand bath of the flowers will calm palpitations, anxiety, and headache. A few drops of the essential oil can be rubbed into the temples during migraine, anxiety attacks and insomnia. The hydrosol is refreshing and soothing. Lavender is bitter and so it stimulates digestion and helps nausea associated with migraine and travel sickness. It can be helpful to alleviate the nausea and side effects of chemotherapy used as an essential oil. Lavender is painkilling, and a strong tea or diluted essential oil is useful for hot heat and redness,

wounds, burns and rashes. To stop a migraine attack, add
15–20 drops of the essential oil to a bath and lie there for
15–20 minutes keeping the water hot. Then lie down in a
darkened room and sleep off the attack. Lavender is one of
the herbs, practitioners use to wean people off tranquillisers
(this must be done under supervision as withdrawal can be
alarming and needs to be carefully managed.) If you wake in
the night, a few drops of lavender essential oil on your pillow or over the heart area will usually send you back into a
deep sleep.

Always do a small patch test with essential oils to check for any
skin sensitivity

Lemon (Citrus x limon)

Lemons need heat and sunshine to grow, and so most of our
lemons come from the southern Mediterranean. I source my
lemons from www.crowdfarming.com. They are organic and
picked a day before shipping.

Part used: the fruit for juice, the rind as a bitter and aromatic
and is added to fire cider and vinegar. After squeezing the
lemon, I cut up the rind and cover it with water (don't do this
with non-organic lemons as the skin is waxed). Drink the next
day; it is incredibly bitter and refreshing. You can also use the
essential oil diluted for wounds and used in steam inhalations.
I use the vinegar as a condiment.

Actions: lemons are an excellent source of Vitamin C. One
lemon provides half our daily requirement (31 mg). Their
anti-inflammatory action has been shown to reduce cholesterol, reduce the incidence of kidney stones, and anaemia (by
increasing iron absorption).

I use lemons as an internal cleansing remedy in spring (one lemon a day for two weeks) and for constipation to build immunity and resit viruses and other pathogens.

Lemons are very acidic. To prevent damage to tooth enamel, be sure to swill your mouth out with water after drinking lemon juice and then clean your teeth

Lemon balm (Melissa officinalis)

Lemon balm grows easily in pots, and in the garden. It is a member of the mint family and spreads like wildfire if not contained. It flowers from June to August.

Part used: the whole plant is used. Melissa is best taken fresh as a tea; boiling water extracts the volatile oils. Otherwise, you can use essential oil or hydrosol or tincture.

Actions: lemon balm is warming, soothing, and mood-elevating. It is the best fresh when you are feeling miserable, lonely, or depressed. Melissa is great digestion for reflux, heartburn, indigestion, and constipation. Use after a meal to help digestion, especially heavy, fatty foods. It stimulates the appetite and is helpful in relaxing the tension, and allows the digestive juices to flow. It helps to remove gas and wind and is used by herbalists to treat ulcers, diverticulitis, and other digestive complaints that are gripping.

Melissa improves circulation and is helpful for high blood pressure due to stress, palpitations, tinnitus, and dizziness.

Linden blossom (Tila europea)

Lime trees blossom in May and June. They are widespread in the UK.

Part used: the strobiles are collected. Lime blossom is taken as a tea and tincture.

Actions: linden blossom is a strong sedative and is used for anxiety, insomnia, and stress. Herbalists use linden blossom for hypertension and to increase artery health. Linden is also useful for panic attacks, palpitations, and to come off the tranquilisers (under supervision). Linden is a great remedy for tension headaches and migraine to lower stress levels and bring on restful sleep.

Linden is used in influenza and for bringing down fevers. Take as a tea. Linden mixes well with peppermint.

Milky oats (Avena sativa)

Milky oats are collected in late summer. They grow wild in country areas; just be sure they are not in a field which has been sprayed with chemicals.

Part used: the milky seed is used and sometimes the oat straw. Milky oats can be taken as a tea, a tincture and as a powder.

Actions: milky oats are nourishment for the nervous system, and so are helpful after shock, mental exhaustion, bereavement and depression.

You can add milky oats to bathwater (put it in a muslin or cotton bag and tie it under the hot tap) to soothe irritated skin, to calm the nerves and relax deeply. If a bath cannot be taken, try a foot bath or hand bath after chemo or other procedure when you feel shocked or upset.

Milk thistle (Silybum marianum)

Milk thistle grows wild, often near the sea, and the seeds are collected in late summer.

Part used: we use the seeds of milk thistle. This is one remedy that is hard to extract, so I recommend you buy the tincture from a reputable supplier. It can be used as a tea and as a powder in capsules.

Actions: milk thistle is a great liver remedy, a bit stronger than calendula. Use where the liver has been stressed, so together with chemotherapy, after accidents and operations, and to support the liver while taking pharmaceuticals. Milk thistle helps with post-viral conditions, acute and chronic infections, poor digestion, constipation, nausea, and varicose veins (from liver congestion).

Mushrooms

We are fortunate in having a super abundance of mushrooms growing wild in the UK. They are collected in the autumn and winter. Ideally, go foraging with an expert the first time.

All mushrooms are edible, but some are only edible once

Turkey tail (Trametes versicolor)

The brightly coloured bracket fungus grows on old, dead wood in shady places, pick in January and February. We use the fruiting body.

Part used: we use the whole mushroom. Mushrooms are best taken as a tincture or powder. Mushrooms need to be double extracted, once in water and afterwards in alcohol. The tea is used in Japan. Turkey tail, reishi and chaga mushrooms are often combined in mushroom coffee.

Actions: Mushrooms are deep acting in the body and so are used in deep-seated chronic diseases. We use turkey tail in chronic infections, during chemotherapy and radiotherapy to recover quicker and reduce side effects. For post-viral conditions, exhaustion or any condition which is deep-seated in the body and has resisted other therapies. Mushrooms are anti-inflammatory and have possible anti-cancer effects; turkey tail is a standard treatment for cancer in Japan and China. It contains prebiotics which support the microbiome, helping the growth of good bacteria, and so is used in leaky gut syndrome (see Nourishment), diverticulitis and other digestive conditions. Turkey Tail is antibacterial, anti-viral and antioxidant and is useful in chronic infections.

Reishi *(*Ganoderma lucidum*)*

It is best to buy reishi from a reputable source; they do grow in the wild, but over-harvesting is rife.

Part used: we use the fruiting body of reishi, which is generally taken as capsules, tincture, or as mushroom coffee; in China, they are added to food and drinks.

Actions: called 'the king of mushrooms' in China, reishi is a superfood. It is anti-inflammatory, immune boosting, and an adaptogen. Adaptogens reduce the effects of stress on the body, namely inflammation, damaged blood vessels (see the chapter on the brain), low energy and vitality (post-viral and ME). Reishi are antioxidants and so help with heart disease, infections, auto-immune conditions, allergies and are possibly cancer protective. They may help with blood sugar levels, improve liver function and chronic, repetitive infections in the bladder and lungs.[146] Reishi may be taken as a supplement as a preventative.

Passiflora *(*Passiflora incarnata*)*

You can grow passiflora in the garden and pick just as the flowers open in summer.

Part used: we use the flowers, leaves, and stem in tea, tincture, or tablets.

Actions: Passiflora is found in many over-the-counter remedies for insomnia, anxiety, and stress. It is often combined with oats (*Avena*) to nourish and heal a depleted nervous system. It is a deep relaxant and stress buster. It is helpful for dizziness and panic attacks.

Sage (Salvia officinalis)

Sage is easily grown in pots and in the garden. It can be picked throughout the summer months.

Part used: the flowers, leaves and stem are used in tea, tinctures, and hydrosol.

Actions: sage is a drying herb and is useful for conditions of fluid build-up in the body. It makes a great mouthwash (as a tea or hydrosol) or as an addition to mouthwashes, and toothpaste and oil-pulling mixtures as an essential oil. Sage is a great remedy for sore throat, hoarseness and tonsilitis. Make a strong tea or put a teaspoon of the tincture in warm water and gargle with it.

Skullcap (Scutelaria latefolia)

You can grow it in the garden, but it is unlikely to be found wild.

Part used: we use the whole herb of skullcap as a tea or tincture.

Actions: skullcap is a relaxant and is often found in sleep mixtures and anti-anxiety mixes. As a tea, it is helpful for headaches and stress. Skullcap is especially useful for the type of insomnia when you wake up in the night and can't get back to sleep in this case drink the tea an hour before retiring or take the tincture three times a day to reset your sleep pattern.

Thyme (Thymus vulgaris)

Thyme flowers throughout the summer months and is easily cultivated as a pot herb.

Part used: we use the flowers and leaves and stem (except for very woody parts). The tea is strong but effective, or the tincture. The essential oil is effective but super strong, so best taken under the supervision of a professional. Add 1 or 2 drops to boiling water to make a good steam inhalation to shift stubborn mucus or get to the root of a bad cough.

Do not take the essential oil internally except under supervision

Actions: thyme is a powerful antiseptic and is a great remedy for both the lungs, mixed with liquorice (see recipes) and for irritated bladder conditions such as cystitis, as a tea mixed with a soothing herb like marshmallow root or corn silk (the fibres from sweet corn). Thyme is strong, do not take for prolonged periods of time, 14 days maximum at one time.

Turmeric (Curcuma longa)

Increasingly turmeric is found in health food shops and can be grown under glass in this country, although I suspect turmeric grown in hot countries has a stronger action.

Part used: the rhizome is used, and it needs fat and pepper to release the active principles, so add a teaspoon of coconut oil or other oil and a few shakes of black pepper when using it fresh in drinks and smoothies. Turmeric is also sold as capsules and tablets (just check they have fat and pepper in them) and all manner of over-the-counter products.

Actions: turmeric has been used for millennia in Indian cooking and medicine for its health-giving qualities. It is anti-inflammatory, and trials have found it useful for inflammatory conditions such as arthritis. It is helpful for heart conditions, is a strong antioxidant and may boost BDNF (see Thinking).

Witch hazel (Hamamelis virginiana)

Witches hazel grows in Northern latitudes; it is a garden plant. It flowers in the winter months.

Part used: we use the bark of witch hazel which is collected in the spring after the flowers have gone.

Actions: witch hazel is usually used externally made into a lotion for varicose veins. It is a strong astringent which reduces the swelling of bruises and leg veins.

Yarrow (Achillea millefolium)

Yarrow grows abundantly in the wild but can also be cultivated.

Part used: we used the whole herb of yarrow, flowers leaves, and stem. It is collected in the late summer months. We use the tea, tincture, essential oil and hydrosol of yarrow.

Actions: yarrow is a strong astringent, and so is useful for wounds and bleeding as a tea or tincture or even the chewed leaves applied onto a wound or up a nostril as a first aid remedy for nosebleeds. Yarrow is anti-inflammatory and is used in infections, especially in the bladder, and it is very helpful for gum problems as a mouthwash, toothpaste and for oil pulling.

Yarrow is one of the herbs used by herbalists to treat circulatory problems and high blood pressure.

Bach flower remedies

These are helpful for emotional states, which then affect the body. Dr Bach categorised the original 38 flower essences he discovered into three categories to assist in their application. The categories are the 12 healers which reflect and transform our essential nature.

- Impatiens. These are irritable people, their minds race ahead, and they have a problem being in the present. They may be lonely as they do not connect well with people.
- Gentian. These people get easily discouraged by setbacks and are often pessimistic about things improving. They may lack self-confidence. Gentian stops feelings of overwhelm and encourages them to persist.
- Mimulus. This is for anxiety and fear. They are empaths or super sensitive to everything and can overact to stress. They are hyper-aroused and have trouble relaxing and sleeping. Mimulus brings calm and courage.
- Clematis. This is for dreamy people who live in their own world. They may have a strong fantasy life and be creative but find everyday tasks hard. They can escape by drinking and TV watching. Clematis brings them back to the present.
- Agrimony. These people hide their suffering behind a façade and have difficulty dealing with deep emotions. They tend to brush off their suffering because they do not know how to express it.
- Chicory. This shows a person who feels very sorry for themselves and feels the victim. They can be demanding and manipulative. They can appear loving, but their care is intended to get attention for themselves. The remedy will allow them to be more selfless.

- Vervain. These people can be bullies, overbearing, and bossy. They are inflexible and often are highly stressed, pushing their bodies to the point of exhaustion. The remedy allows them to embrace softness and flexibility.
- Centaury. These people who can be 'doormats' and lack strong boundaries. They have a poor sense of their own self-worth and can be used and abused by other people. Chicory builds self-esteem and boundaries.
- Scleranthus. These are people who are hesitant and confused. They hate making decisions and get very upset by their indecisiveness. They can dwell on choices and become exhausted at all the choices open to them. Scleranthus helps them to build an inner sense of knowing.
- Water violet. This opens the heart of people who are cut off from their feelings and who avoid intimacy with others. The remedy helps them to open up to love and companionship.
- Rock rose. This is for panic and terror, especially big shocks or life traumas like a terminal diagnosis, sudden death, or accident. It helps with the fear of dying and brings courage and some detachment. Rock rose is a component of Rescue Remedy.
- Cerato. This is for people who do not trust their own feelings and intuition. They constantly ask other people to decide for them, and they cannot hear their own inner wisdom. Cerato develops trust in their own inner knowing.

Herbalist organisations

National Institute of Medical Herbalists – https://nimh. org.uk/

The College of Practitioners of Phytotherapy – www.ccp.uk

Association of Master Herbalists – www.associationofmaster-herbalists.co.uk

Unified Register of Herbal Practitioners – www.urhp.com

American Herbalists Guild – www.americanherbalistsguild.com

The Herb Society promotes the use of herbs – www.herbsociety.org.uk

Herbal remedy suppliers

For herbs, tinctures, essential oils, etc.

www.caleysapothecary.co.uk

www.Baldwins.co.uk

For oils, waxes, and ingredients to make creams and lotions – www.Aromantic.co.uk

For high-quality hydrosols and essential oils – www.Oshadi.co.uk

For mushrooms – www.myconutri.com

Books

Aeon Books has a variety of books on herbs – www.aeonbooks.co.uk

Herb growing and tincture making: Lucy Jones. *Self-Sufficient Herbalism*. Aeon.

Making creams and ointments: Dawn Ireland. *Herbal Cream Making*. Herbary Books.

Action

Practical information

General wellness vlogs and podcasts:

https://zdoggmd.com

www.drhyman.com

www.drchatterjee.com

www.onecommune.com

www.patrickholford.com

They all produce newsletters and vlogs and record interviews with experts in their fields which are accessible to lay people.

Chapter 1: Nourishment

Professor Tim Spector[147] suggests five things to do to improve our nourishment for body, mind, and emotions.

1. Eat the rainbow.
Every week eat 30 different coloured vegetables and fruits. He includes nuts and seeds here.

Here is a small list:

Red: strawberries, red peppers, red chilli, red onions, red cabbage, aubergine, tomatoes, kidney beans, aduki beans, apples, raspberries, and beetroot.

Orange: turmeric, mango, papaya, orange peppers, oranges, carrots, swede, sweet potatoes, orange (red) lentils, apricots, peaches, grapefruit.

Yellow: bananas, pineapple, garlic, chickpeas, yellow lentils, lemons, grapefruit, cashew nuts, ginger, honeydew melon, avocados, squash, sweetcorn.

White: lychees, white cabbage, cannelloni beans, white miso, cauliflower, cucumber, fennel, celery, kiwis, pears,

Blue: blackberries, blueberries, loganberries, blackcurrants, grapes,

Green: kale, spinach, Brussel sprouts, cabbage, broccoli, cavolo nero, peas, watercress, lettuce, green beans, French beans, all salad greens, leeks, spring greens, herbs like coriander, mint, parsley, thyme, rosemary, sage etc. courgettes,

Brown: mushrooms, Brazil nuts, brown onions,

2. Rest your gut.
Leave 12–14 hours between your last food in the evening and breakfast.

3. Eat fermented foods.
Kimchi, miso, piccalilli, any foods which have been fermented, and cheese also come into this category.

4. Avoid highly processed foods.
Pre-packaged meals, takeaways, anything with ingredients you cannot identity and would not normally have at home. Save these for occasional treats, high days, and holidays.

5. Eat at least 30 different kinds of fruit and vegetable during a week.

Good food suppliers

Organic food is best, or freshly picked from Farmers' markets or farm shops.

Veg-boxes are an ideal way to get a good variety of vegetables in season, and as a bonus it keeps you out of supermarkets where temptation may lie!

www.riverford.co.uk

www.abelandcole.co.uk

Within the M25 and Kent – www.kentvegbox.com

Many supermarkets now sell some organic produce; go for those on the 'dirty dozen list' if funds are limited.

Pesticides: the dirty dozen[148] and the clean 15 list

The foods with the most pesticides and those with the least, which are ok to eat non-organic. The list is from the US, but it is likely levels are similar in the UK. The list is updated every year.

Dirty dozen (worst first)—Clean 15 (best first)

* Strawberries – Avocados
* Spinach – Sweet corn
* Kale – Pineapple
* Nectarines – Onions
* Apples – Papaya
* Grapes – Peas (frozen)
* Bell pepper – Asparagus
* Cherries – Honeydew melon
* Peaches – Kiwi

- Pears   –   Cabbage
- Celery   –   Mushrooms
- Tomatoes   –   Cantaloupe
- Mango
- Watermelon
- Sweet potato

Superfoods (see the chapter on Nourishment and section on Methylation for details)

Seaweeds, mushrooms (especially shiitake), turmeric, garlic, lemons, berries, seeds, green tea.

Polyphenols

Green tea, coffee, berries, vegetables such as artichokes, olives, and asparagus.

Cooking ideas

I have found BBC Food (www.bbcfood.com) has consistently good recipes suitable for beginners and experienced cooks.

The Mindful Chef (www.themindfulchef.co.uk) has great vegan recipes and also does recipe boxes, as does Riverford. Recipe boxes, where all the ingredients are collected together with a recipe, offer a good way to gain confidence in cooking.

Zoe

Zoe is a project run by Professor Tim Spector (www.joinzoe. com) in collaboration with Kings College London, Stanford Medicine, Harvard School of Public Health, and Massachusetts General Hospital, where participants are monitored for gut bacteria, blood sugar, and blood fats. These are measured via a kit, and a personalised nutritional programme is developed for participants, and everyone reacts differently to foods. It is pricey but gives a personalised picture of your health and how you respond to food which can be used forever more.

Foraging: picking your own food from the countryside and learning how to cook it (www.foragers-association.org)

Chapter 2: Rest

Breathing exercises

The 478 breathing technique

This technique activates the diaphragm through deep belly breathing, which stimulates the vagus nerve and stops adrenal overactivity, and calms the mind and body.

- Exhale completely through the mouth to activate the diaphragm.
- Inhale, close your eyes and count to 4.
- Visualise breath travelling up to your eyes.
- Place the tip of your tongue on the roof of your mouth, and expand your abdomen.
- Hold for seven counts.
- Exhale via mouth for eight counts. This massages the diaphragm and calms down the central nervous system (CNS).
- Do this for four cycles, twice a day, once during the day and once one hour before bedtime.

The 48 breathing technique

- If you wake during the night, inhale for four counts and exhale for eight counts.
- This calms the CNS, and the mind will disengage from thinking as all your awareness is focused on the breath. As you breathe, have no expectation or attachment to any result.
- Alternate nostrils.

- Close one nostril with the thumb and breathe through the other one.
- Count to 6 breathing in and 6 breathing out. Do this ten times on each side (count with your fingers on the other hand). This brings air to the brain and allows both hemispheres of the brain to become balanced. If you are stressed during the day, this practice calms your CNS.

Snoring

3M micropore surgical tape.

Environmental toxins

Environmental toxins affect our immune system and can cause inflammation in the whole body. Avoid, xenoestrogens, or EDCs (endocrine disruptive compounds),[149] which are environmental toxins and believed to disrupt hormones, including the thyroid. They are found in nature, are healthy, and include BPA found in plastics (including food containers), PFAs found in non-stick pans and textiles, and phthalates found in packaging, cosmetics, and medical devices. Try to use natural skin care (or make your own, see Materia Medica for recipes), eat organic foods see above, use natural cleaning agents such as vinegar and bicarbonate of soda rather than harsh chemicals, and try not to store food in plastics, avoid cling film and unnecessary packaging.

If you are suffering from a serious inflammatory condition, consider if you come in contact with the following:

- Pharmaceutical drugs.
- Mould.
- Heavy metals such as mercury and lead, etc.

Sixty per cent of lipsticks have lead in them so check your products. Think Dirty (https://thinkdirtyapp.com) is an app you can put on your phone to check the chemicals in foods, etc.

Check your mattress; use futons or other good quality mattresses. VOCs (volatile organic compounds)[150] are everywhere and are found in higher concentrations inside the home. VOCs can be found in paint, carpets, air fresheners, candles, cosmetics, cleaning products, dry cleaning fumes, and flame retardants. VOCs are toxic to susceptible people; use organic pillows and sheets, and try sleeping with an open window. It can take up to seven years to 'off-gas' VOCs in the home.

Car interiors take eight months to 'off gas'. The best way to remove the most VOCs in new cars is to park in the sunshine with the windows closed. The heat draws the toxins out of the materials, then leave the car with open doors once a week or drive with the windows open. These solvents cross the blood-brain barrier and may cause fatigue, brain fog, headaches and waking up with a 'drunk feeling'.

For any VOCs, fresh air is your friend, have open windows, where possible. Saunas help to detoxify the body, and charcoal (available as tablets) binds the solvents, so they are not reabsorbed.

Cruciferous vegetables, avocado, garlic, and onions help to clear the body, as well as taking liver, kidney, and lymphatic herbs to clear the body such as calendula, dandelion herb and root, cleavers etc (see Materia Medica).

For a list of volatile organic compounds see www.thefiltery. com/volatile-organic-compounds-vocs-list/

How to meditate without meditating[151]

This was the title of an interesting article in the *Guardian* newspaper, which gave alternative suggestions for chilling out and re-invigorating the mind. Here are a few of them, but do read the article for the whole picture.

- The aim of meditation is to bring your awareness back into the present moment, and attempt to stay in the moment, allowing thoughts, emotions, and feelings to pass by without comment.
- This state can be achieved by being in nature. Nature brings about a sense of awe; remember the broad horizons on top of hills or mountains, the beauty of sunsets or dappled sunshine through a shady wood. Nature causes us to pause, to drink in space, beauty, and timelessness and can put all our concerns into perspective. Looking a nature rests the eyes and stills the mind.
- Being in the flow is a meditative state, whether it is model making, gardening, cooking or cleaning, or doing creative activities like drawing, painting, dressmaking, or knitting. They will all calm the thoughts, and you can soon zoom out. Listening to music or making music has the same effect as does writing, anything where we 'lose ourselves'.
- I am a great fan of doing nothing. Staring out of the window, watching the birds in the sky, or trees blow in the wind. We don't do enough of nothing; it can be a super relaxing, meditative state. Turn off those devices and allow yourself half an hour to simply be, notice thoughts and feelings and let them do.

Learning meditation

There are lots of places and methods of meditation available, depending on your preferences. I like these London Mindful (www.londonmindful.com/) as they have drop-in sessions online, which are by donation.

Chapter 3: Stretch

Yin yoga

Mel Skinner, author of *Rest is Radical*,[152] gives online classes – http://www.melskinneryoga.com/online-classes

Online exercise classes

Sophie Butler, a wheelchair-bound instructor, is friendly and accessible – www.youtube.com/watch?v=BvXti5fgtBQ

Mike Kutcher exercise videos aimed at the over 60s – www.youtube.com/c/MoreLifeHealth

Yoga videos abound on YouTube. The instructors I favour are Kino McGregor and Laruga; both teach Ashtanga, which is a dynamic practice – www.youtube.com/@KinoYoga and www.youtube.com/@larugayoga

Indaba Yoga (https://indabayoga.com/) is based in London but do online courses.

Outdoor exercises

Run, walk, or monitor. These runs are available throughout the country – www.parkrun.org.uk

Countrywide groups who walk the countryside – www.ramblers.org.uk

For those more inclined to amble – https://beta.ramblers.org.uk/go-walking/wellbeing-walks

The Ramblers website says:

> Fitness level doesn't matter. Walks are over easy terrain and at a steady pace to suit everyone.
>
> Mobility limitations aren't an issue: routes are open to all (Please contact the walk organiser to check if the route is wheelchair accessible).
>
> No special equipment is needed.
>
> Wellbeing walks are achievable: walks are short: starting at ten minutes and never longer than 90 minutes.
>
> Making walking a healthy habit is easier: there's at least one planned walk a week, starting at the same time and place every week.

Finding a Ramblers Wellbeing Walk is simple: planned walks feature on our website.

Joining a group walk is convenient: all walks are local, and accessible on foot or by public transport.

Walking in a group keeps your motivation high and offers the possibility of making new friends.

Chapter 4: Thinking

Life on a Knife's Edge: A Brain Surgeon's Reflections on Life, Loss, and Survival, by Rahul Jandial, 2021. London: Penguin Life.

Life Lessons from a Brain Surgeon: The New Science and Stories of the Brain, by Rahul Jandial, 2019. London: Penguin Life.

Tara Brach offers a variety of meditations on her website, pay by donation – www.tarabrach.com/guided-meditations/

Exercise that brain at Headway (https://headway-product. com/start), who offer (for a fee) 15-minute bite-sized extracts of books, both fiction and non-fiction.

Adult education: offers a myriad of courses to stretch the brain

University of the Third Age (www.U3A.org) offers local groups plus online courses.

Check your brain health at Food for the Brain (https://foodforthebrain.org/), who aim to do this yearly to keep an eye on things.

Chapter 5: Happiness

Psychedelics

There is a great deal of interest in psychedelics for mental health. Psilocybin is illegal in the UK, but clinical trials are happening in Manchester and Kings College London on its use for patients with treatment-resistant depression.

Alberts Labs (https://albertlabs.com) are conducting research, as are Clerkenwell Health (www.clerkenwellhealth.com).

There are groups in Holland who do work with psychedelics – www.alalaho.org

The Psychedelic Network (https://psychedelicnetwork.org.uk/) also has a list of retreats and practitioners who work with psychedelics and a newsletter on the latest research.

The Psychedelic Society has lots of info on its website and runs a wide variety of workshops and courses, and videos at www.psychedelicsociety.org.uk.

For training and events around the therapeutic use of psychedelics – https://instituteofpsychedelictherapy.org

Meditation

There are lots of meditations online. Check out:

www.Tarabrachcom

www.deepakchopra.com

For online courses and drop-in sessions – www.londonmindful.com/

Grief

Cariad Lloyd has a great podcast on grief – https://cariadlloyd.com/griefcast

For online grief counsellors and lots of resources for living with grief – www.cruse.org.uk/

For lots of resources and a phone line for support – www.mariecurie.org.uk/help/support/bereavement

Help

The Samaritans (www.samaritans.org/) can be contacted via the phone, text, email, or snail-mail, and some of the larger offices have 1:1 sessions. All free.

Age Concern (www.ageuk.org.uk/) offer phone helplines and a befriending service.

Chapter 6: Connection

Kindness

How kind are you? The kindness test measures this – www.testmykindness.org/

Helping others

Befriend an older, isolated person – www.ageuk.org.uk

Help literacy by reading with schoolchildren – www.schoolreaders.org/volunteer and www.beanstalkcharity.org.uk. Do this online at www.bookmarkreading.org

Foster an animal for people who are sick or cannot walk their animals or take them to the vet – www.rspca.org.uk

Be a mentor in the arts – www.artsemergency.org.uk

Be a mentor in the tech sector – www.meetamentor.co.uk

Mentor a child in London – www.bigbrothersbigsistersuk.org

Mentor a child in Manchester – www.reachoutuk.org

Gig Buddies (www.gigbuddies.org) match up people to accompany an autistic person to gigs and other events to help them navigate public space and crowds.

Knit for charity (www.prima.co.uk). Your local neonatal ward might well need baby booties and hats for the newborn.

Become a trustee of a local charity. They are often looking for people with a variety of skillsets – reachvolunteering.org.uk

Support your local food bank. The Trussell Trust has volunteer opportunities – https://volunteer.trusselltrust.org/

Help refugees (www.care4calais.org) by donating clothes. You can also volunteer in the UK and in Calais, fundraising and campaign opportunities are available.

Find an organisation which represents a special interest, trees, trains, or travel and network or volunteer there. There are too many to list all of them (this shows how we are really social animals). Here are a few:

Community spaces for men to connect, converse and create. The activities are often similar to those of garden sheds, but for groups of men to enjoy together. They help reduce loneliness and isolation, but most importantly, they're fun – https://menssheds.org.uk/

Men Without Masks offer men's retreats and a network to support all men in a safe environment – www.menwithoutmasks.com

Knit and natter groups – www.ageuk.org and www.ukhand-knitting.com/

Walking groups include short walks for all, many wheelchair accessible – https://beta.ramblers.org.uk/go-walking/wellbeing-walks

Foraging groups: lists, walks, and courses – https://foragers-association.org and www.countryfile.com/how-to/foraging/best-foraging-courses-in-uk

Learning to make herbal remedies and supporting homeless communities in London – www.phytology.org/apothecary

Writing groups, most adult education institutes offer creative writing courses. National Writing Project UK lists groups throughout the country – www.nationalwritingproject.uk/writing-groups

Exercise groups – www.ageuk.org.uk/services/in-your-area

This website has more details – www.compassionate-communities...

Listen

Dr Julian's Podcast – Survival of the Kindest – www.compassionate-communities...

Podcast with Dr Julian Abel – https://drchatterjee.com/the-healing-power-of-compassion-with-dr-julian-abel

TED talk Compassion Matters, Julian Abel – www.ted.com/talks/dr_julian_abel_why_compassion_matters

TED talk Joan Halifax on compassion and empathy – www.ted.com/talks/joan_halifax_compassion_and_the_true_meaning_of_empathy

Chapter 7: Fun

Reading: join a book club or start your own – www.booksclubs.com

Wine:
www.seachangewine.com – some organic wines, ethical company.

www.dryfarmwines.com – ethical, organic, sugar free wines from small wineries

www.theorganicsommelier.co.uk – sustainable, organic, vegan wines.

Chocolate:
www.cocoaloco.com – fairtrade, organic and vegan chocolate.

www.wearefairtrade.com – chocolate and other fairtrade products including coffee.

Oxfam shops sell, fairtrade and organic chocolate: Tony's and Divine brands.

Co-Op supermarkets and Waitrose sell fairtrade organic chocolate.

www.hotelchocolat.com – vegan and fairtrade chocolate.

Coffee:
www.cafedirect.co.uk – fairtrade coffee in Oxfam shops and supermarkets.

www.yallahcoffee.co.uk – carbon neutral coffee, arrives by sail direct from growers.

www.oddcoffeeco.com – 'rescue' coffee pods, ground coffee and coffee beans.

Music:
Many music schools have free concerts for their pupils to showcase their talent. Churches and libraries often have music at lunchtimes. Check your local listings.

Dancing:
www.ageuk.org.uk – countrywide listings for over 60s activities including dance.

Ecstatic dancing is free dancing to trance music and sessions are alcohol free and open to all ages – www.ecstaticdance.org www.ecstaticdancelondon.com

Tea dances: check out www.meetup.com for local groups.

For contemporary dances classes in London for the over 60s – www.artsdepot.co.uk and www.theplace.org.uk – www.rambert.org.uk – www.eastlondondance.org. Check local dance schools and dance troupes for classes.

Sex: used by adult women of all ages, and we're really keen to foreground and normalise all under representations of consensual sexual pleasure.

Listen

Boyce, C. (2023). 'I've spent years studying happiness – here's what actually makes for a happier life'. *The Conversation* – https://theconversation.com/ive-spent-years-studying-happiness-heres-what-actually-makes-for-a-happier-life-197580

Chapter 8: Checking out

Psychedelics and the end of life

One thing that psychedelics offer us is an opportunity to re-evaluate our lives and make peace with ourselves and others. Psilocybin is illegal in the UK. But clinical trials are happening in Manchester and Kings College London on its use for patients with a terminal diagnosis.

There are groups in Holland who do work with psychedelics – www.alalaho.org

The Psychedelic Network (https://psychedelicnetwork.org.uk/) also has a list of retreats and practitioners who work with psychedelics and a newsletter on the latest research.

The Psychedelic Society has lots of info on its website and runs a wide variety of workshops and courses and videos – www.psychedelicsociety.org.uk.

For training and events around the therapeutic use of psychedelics – https://instituteofpsychedelictherapy.org

Links and contacts

Natural Death campaigns for dignity in dying – www.nat-
uraldeath.org.uk

The Death Cafe website gives lists of nearby Death Cafe meet-
ings – www.thedeathcafe.com.

Soul Midwives provide lists of Soul Midwives and lots of info
on their work and gentle dying – www.soulmidwives.co.uk

Death Doulas do similar work to Soul Midwives – www.death-
doulas.com

Compassion in Dying campaign for control over the dying
process – https://compassionindying.org.uk/

Dignity in Dying campaigns for the legalisation of assisted
dying in the UK – www.dignityindying.org.uk

Essence Medicine use non-psychedelic processes working with
psycho-spiritual care for people with a terminal diagnosis, and
trainings for professionals. Essence is run by a doctor and hospice nurse. Essence offers online groups and retreats for people
with a terminal diagnosis. They offer some bursaries – www.
essence_medicine.com

Penny Brohn offers many resources for those will a cancer/
terminal diagnosis – www.pennybrohn.org.uk/ previously the
Bristol Cancer centre

Books

Elizabeth Kubler-Ross. *On Death and Dying*. 1969. London:
Macmillan.

Felicity Warner. *Sacred Oils*. 2022. London: Hay House.

Felicity Warner. *A Safe Journey Home*. 2011. London: Hay House.

Bonnie Ware. *Top Five Regrets of the Dying*. 2019. London: Hay House.

Raymond Moody. *Life After Life*. 2022. London: Rider.

Films

Dosed on psychedelics and mental health and dying About a woman with a terminal diagnosis who takes psychedelics – www.dosedmovie.com

TED talk Roland Griffiths PhD Johns Hopkins University. *The Science of Psychedelics and it used to relieve suffering* – www.youtube.com/watch?v=AT26zYc9HPg

ENDNOTES

1. There are many, including Dr Mark Hyman, Dr Chatterjee, ZDogg MD, and Zack Bush MD.
2. You can buy home testing glucose monitors if you wish to isolate which foods trigger an insulin response in you. Join Zoe, www.joinzoe.com, is running a project to test our individual glucose response.
3. Re-evaluation of the traditional diet-heart hypothesis: analysis of recovered data from Minnesota Coronary Experiment (1968–1973). April 2016. www.bmj.com/content/353/bmj.i1246
4. An interesting series of articles on health, diet, and chronic disease – www.jeffnobbs.com/posts/what-causes-chronic-disease
5. http://ash.org.uk/wp-content/uploads/2016/06/Smoking-Statistics-Who-Smokes-and-How-Much.pdf
6. www.jeffnobbs.com/posts/what-causes-chronic-disease
7. www.jeffnobbs.com/posts/what-causes-chronic-disease
8. www.jeffnobbs.com/posts/what-causes-chronic-disease
9. Alice Park, 'When vegetable oil isn't as healthy as you think'. *Time Magazine*, 12 April 2016. https://time.com/4291505/when-vegetable-oil-isnt-as-healthy-as-you-think/
10. A. Bacyinski, M. Xu, W. Wang, and J. Hu. (2017) 'The paravascular pathway for brain waste clearance: Current understanding, significance and controversy'. *Frontiers in*

Neuroanatomy, 11: 101. https://doi.org/10.3389/fnana.2017. 00101. PMC 5681909. PMID 29163074.

11. https://web.archive.org/web/20080124000744/www.help-guide.org/life/sleeping.htm

12. A. Fry. (9 October 2020). *Napping: Health Benefits & Tips for your Best Nap.* Sleep Foundation – www.sleepfoundation.org/ sleep-hygiene/napping.

13. S.M. Schmid, M. Hallschmid, and B. Schultes. (January 2015) 'The metabolic burden of sleep loss'. *The Lancet. Diabetes & Endocrinology*, 3 (1): 52–62. https://doi.org/10.1016/ S2213-8587(14)70012-9

14. da Silveira, Matheus Pelinski et al. (2021) 'Physical exercise as a tool to help the immune system against COVID-19: an integrative review of the current literature'. *Clinical and Experimental Medicine*, 21 (1): 15–28. https://doi.org/10.1007/ s10238-020-00650-3

15. Lance Bollinger and Tom LaFontaine. (2011) 'Exercise Programming For Insulin Resistance'. *Strength and Conditioning Journal*, 3: 44–47. https://doi.org/10.1519/SSC.0b013e31822599fb

16. https://pubmed.ncbi.nlm.nih.gov/29775542/

17. Physical inactivity is also associated with many chronic conditions (Lee et al., 2012), a reduction in executive function (Daly et al., 2014; Peven et al., 2018), premature mortality (Carlson et al., 2018) as well as increased risk of dementia and Alzheimer's disease (Aarsland et al., 2010; Laurin et al., 2001). In a clinical setting, beneficial effects of physical fitness interventions on cognitive performance have been reported in older persons (Peig-Chiello et al., 1998; Satoh et al., 1995). Epidemiological studies have also reported that exercise may be protective for dementia and Alzheimer's disease in older populations (Laurin et al., 2001; Li et al., 1989).

    Silvin P. Knight et al. (2012) 'Obesity is associated with reduced cerebral blood flow – modified by physical activity'. *Neurobiology of Aging*, 105: 35–47. https://doi. org/10.1016/j.neurobiolaging.2021.04.008.

    www.ncbi.nlm.nih.gov/pmc/articles/PMC8600128/?_ kx=4S-Imp1QFt-VFhFZopFyW2tT3P-wUeGKB6M0V_I4ZGP-xcOLBAwUC71NoegX8Cgc.HKMsXE accessed 6 January 2023.

18. C.L. Craig, A.L. Marshall, M. Sjöström, A.E. Bauman, M.L. Booth, B.E. Ainsworth, M. Pratt, U. Ekelund, A. Yngve, J.F. Sallis, and P. Oja. (2003) 'International physical activity questionnaire: 12-country reliability and validity'. *Med. Sci. Sports. Exerc.*, 35: 1381–1395.
19. www.omnicalculator.com/sports/met-minutes-per-week#met-definition
20. https://bjsm.bmj.com/content/56/17/975
21. www.ncbi.nlm.nih.gov/pmc/articles/PMC6323335/
22. www.theguardian.com/lifeandstyle/2022/oct/30/walk-nature-good-for-mind-body-soul?fbclid=IwAR2lxO3EEFd0wwo-6h1Ca96gR2vhhby9pqY3UZyNz9TTuBQsovWmQGBS5pA.

    Jessica Lee. 'Giant Steps: why walking in nature is good for mind, body, and soul'. *The Guardian*, 30 October 2022.
23. I. Lee, E.J. Shiroma, M. Kamada, D.R. Bassett, C.E. Matthews, and J.E. Buring. (2019) 'Association of Step Volume and Intensity With All-Cause Mortality in Older Women'. *JAMA Intern Med*, 179.8: 1105–1112. https://doi.org/10.1001/jamainternmed.2019.0899
24. Del Pozo Cruz, Borja et al. (2022) 'How many steps a day to reduce the risk of all-cause mortality? A dose-response meta-analysis'. *Journal of Internal Medicine*, 291 (4): 519–521. doi:10.1111/joim.13413
25. R.S. Ulrich. (1984) 'View through a window may influence recovery from surgery'. *Science*, 224.4647: 420–421.
26. J. Pretty, J. Peacock, M. Sellens, and M. Griffin. (2005) 'The mental and physical health outcomes of green exercise'. *Int J Environ Health Res.*, 15.5: 319–337. https://doi.org/10.1080/09603120500155963. PMID: 16416750.
27. M. Polley, M. Bertotti, R. Kimberlee, K. Pilkington, and C. Refsum. (2017) 'A review of the evidence assessing impact of social prescribing on healthcare demand and cost implications'. University of Westminster, 2017. https://westminsterresearch.westminster.ac.uk/item/q1455/a-review-of-the-evidence-assessing-impact-of-social-prescribing-on-healthcare-demand-and-cost-implications
28. www.parkrun.org.uk
29. www.youtube.com/channel/UCtcIcjW5VMQdoqqc MGdrgkw

30. H. Poikonen, P. Toiviainen, and M. Tervaniemi. (2018) 'Naturalistic music and dance: Cortical phase synchrony in musicians and dancers'. *PLoS ONE* 13.4: e0196065. https://doi.org/10.1371/journal.pone.0196065

31. S. Kramer, 'How Busting Some Moves on the Dancefloor is Good for Your Brain'. *New Scientist*, 18 December 2018.

32. Maxine Campion and Liat Levita. (2014) 'Enhancing positive affect and divergent thinking abilities: Play some music and dance'. *The Journal of Positive Psychology*, 9 (2): 137–145. https://doi.org/10.1080/17439760.2013.848376

33. Agnieszka Z. Burzynska, Yuqin Jiao, Anya M. Knecht, Jason Fanning, Elizabeth A. Awick, Tammy Chen, Neha Gothe, Michelle W. Voss, Edward McAuley, and Arthur F. Kramer. (2017) 'White Matter integrity declined over 6-months, but dance intervention improved integrity of the fornix of older adults'. *Frontiers in Aging Neuroscience*, 9: 2017. www.frontiersin.org/articles/10.3389/fnagi.2017.00059.

34. https://drchatterjee.com/bitesize-life-lessons-from-a-brain-surgeon-dr-rahul-jandial/ www.drchattergee.com

35. Docosahexaenoic acid is an Omega 3 fatty acid that is a primary structural component of the human brain, cerebral cortex, skin, and retina. It is found in breast milk, fatty fish, and marine algae.

36. There is lots of research and claims for MCT oil, check out the scientific research here: www.healthline.com/nutrition/mct-oil-benefits

37. I. Anjum, S.S. Jaffery, M. Fayyaz, Z. Samoo, and S. Anjum. (2018) 'The Role of Vitamin D in Brain Health: A Mini Literature Review'. *Cureus*, 10 (7): e2960. https://doi.org/10.7759/cureus.2960

38. I. Anjum, S.S. Jaffery, M. Fayyaz, Z. Samoo, and S. Anjum. (2018) 'The Role of Vitamin D in Brain Health: A Mini Literature Review'. *Cureus*, 10 (7): e2960. https://doi.org/10.7759/cureus.2960v

39. I. Anjum, S.S. Jaffery, M. Fayyaz, Z. Samoo, and S. Anjum. (2018) 'The Role of Vitamin D in Brain Health: A Mini Literature Review'. *Cureus*, 10 (7): e2960. https://doi.org/10.7759/cureus.2960

40. I. Anjum, S.S. Jaffery, M. Fayyaz, Z. Samoo, and S. Anjum. (2018) 'The Role of Vitamin D in Brain Health: A Mini Literature Review'. *Cureus*, 10 (7): e2960. https://doi.org/10.7759/cureus.2960

41. K.N. Fitzgerald, R. Hodges, D. Hanes, E. Stack, D. Cheishvili, M. Szyf, J. Henkel, M.W. Twedt, D. Giannopoulou, J. Herdell, S. Logan, and R. Bradley. (2021) 'Potential reversal of epigenetic age using a diet and lifestyle intervention: a pilot randomized clinical trial'. *Aging*, 13: 9419–9432. https://doi.org/10.18632/aging.202913

42. Methyltetrahydrofolate reductase (MTHFR), catechol-O-methyltransferase (COMT), and cystathione beta-synthase (CBS) – https://wholisticmatters.com/food-nutrition-methylation

43. Adiv A. Johnson et al. (2012) 'The role of DNA methylation in aging, rejuvenation, and age-related disease'. *Rejuvenation Research*, 15.5: 483–494. https://doi.org/10.1089/rej.2012.1324

44. J.M. Sedivy, G. Banumathy, and P.D. Adams. (2012) 'Aging by epigenetics – a consequence of chromatin damage?' *Exp Cell Res.*, 314: 1909–1917. In Adiv A. Johnson et al. 'The role of DNA methylation in aging, rejuvenation, and age-related disease'. *Rejuvenation Research*, 15.5: 483–494. https://doi.org/10.1089/rej.2012.1324

45. Frank Lyko. (2017) 'The DNA methyltransferase family: a versatile toolkit for epigenetic regulation'. *Nature reviews. Genetics*, 19.2: 81–92. https://doi.org/10.1038/nrg.2017.80

46. https://wholisticmatters.com/food-nutrition-methylation

47. I. Onakpoya, E. Spencer, M. Thompson et al. (2014) 'The effect of chlorogenic acid on blood pressure: A systematic review and meta-analysis of randomized clinical trials'. *J Hum Hypertens*, 29: 77–81. https://doi.org/10.1038/jhh.2014.46 and www.nutritionadvance.com/chlorogenic-acid-health-benefits/

48. K.N. Fitzgerald, R. Hodges, D. Hanes, E. Stack, D. Cheishvili, M. Szyf, J. Henkel, M.W. Twedt, D. Giannopoulou, J. Herdell, S. Logan, and R. Bradley. (2021) 'Potential reversal of epigenetic age using a diet and lifestyle intervention: a pilot randomized clinical trial'. *Aging*, 13: 9419–9432. www.aging-us.com/article/202913/text and https://doi.org/10.18632/aging.202913.

49. Methyltetrahydrofolate reductase (MTHFR), catechol-O-methyltransferase (COMT), and cystathione beta-synthase (CBS) – https://wholisticmatters.com/food-nutrition-methylation

50. Adiv A. Johnson et al. (2012) 'The role of DNA methylation in aging, rejuvenation, and age-related disease'. *Rejuvenation Research*, 15 (5): 483–494. https://doi.org/10.1089/rej.2012.1324

51. J.M. Sedivy, G. Banumathy, and P.D. Adams. (2008) 'Aging by epigenetics – a consequence of chromatin damage?' *Exp Cell Res.*, 314: 1909–1917. In Adiv A. Johnson et al. (2012) 'The role of DNA methylation in aging, rejuvenation, and age-related disease'. *Rejuvenation Research*, 15.5: 483–494. https://doi.org/10.1089/rej.2012.1324

52. K.N. Fitzgerald, R. Hodges, D. Hanes, E. Stack, D. Cheishvili, M. Szyf, J. Henkel, M.W. Twedt, D. Giannopoulou, J. Herdell, S. Logan, and R. Bradley. (2021) 'Potential reversal of epigenetic age using a diet and lifestyle intervention: a pilot randomized clinical trial'. *Aging*, 13: 9419–9432. https://doi.org/10.18632/aging.202913.

    Methylation is a constantly changing process in our cells which responds to dietary and environmental factors (epigenetics) and affects gene expression in the body.

53. Andrew Octavian Sasmita. (2019) 'Modification of the gut microbiome to combat neurodegeneration'. *Reviews in the Neurosciences* 30.8: 795–805. https://doi.org/10.1515/revneuro-2019-0005

54. N.M. Vogt, R.L. Kerby, K.A. Dill-McFarland et al. (2017) 'Gut microbiome alterations in Alzheimer's disease'. *Sci Rep*, 7: 13537. https://doi.org/10.1038/s41598-017-13601-y

55. A case history of reducing Alzheimer's symptoms using diet and vitamins from Food for the Brain Foundation – https://foodforthebrain.org/ive-got-my-husband-back-thanks-to-cognition/?utm_source=sendinblue&utm_campaign=Nodge%20and%20Dorothy%20Case%20Study%20-%20to%20CFT%20users%20180323&utm_medium=email

56. www.scientificamerican.com/article/is-it-true-that-creativit/

57. N. Hawkes. (2018) 'Pfizer abandons research into Alzheimer's and Parkinson's diseases'. *BMJ*, 360: k122. doi:10.1136/bmj.k122

58. https://alzheimersprevention.org/downloadables/ FINGER-study-report-by-ARPF.pdf
59. Richard E. Kennedy et al. (2018) 'Association of Concomitant Use of Cholinesterase Inhibitors or Memantine With Cognitive Decline in Alzheimer Clinical Trials: A Meta-analysis'. *JAMA Network Open*, 1.7: e184080. https://doi.org/10.1001/jamanetworkopen.2018.4080
60. Debora Mackenzie. 'We may finally know what causes Alzheimer's – and how to stop it'. *New Scientist*, 23 January 2019, updated 30 January 2019.
61. See David Perlmutter and Austin Permutter. *Brain Wash*. 2020.London: Little Brown, p. 36 for the case of Mr Gage who damaged his brain and his emotional responses altered dramatically.
62. https://news.yale.edu/2021/07/05/psychedelic-spurs-growth-neural-connections-lost-depression
63. https://discovery.ucl.ac.uk/id/eprint/10039986/
64. ww2.kiyumi.org/gabor-mate/
65. www.newscientist.com/article/2149489-different-meditation-types-train-distinct-parts-of-your-brain/
66. www.ncbi.nlm.nih.gov/pmc/articles/PMC1361002/
67. www.ncbi.nlm.nih.gov/pmc/articles/PMC8229690/
68. www.ncbi.nlm.nih.gov/pmc/articles/PMC8229690/
69. www.theguardian.com/media/2013/apr/12/news-is-bad-rolf-dobelli
70. www.statista.com/statistics/898353/daily-audiovisual-viewing-time-by-device-uk/
71. Rolf Dobelli. *The Art of the Good life*. 2017. London: Sceptre.
72. Meta-data studies on HPFs and mental illness – www.ncbi.nlm.nih.gov/pmc/articles/PMC9268228/
73. Matt Haig. *Reasons to Stay Alive*. 2016. London: Canongate,.
74. Dorotyh Rowe. *Depression: The Way Out of Your Prison*. 2003. London: Routledge.
75. 'What we should all know about depression'. 16 August 2010 – hwww.dorothyrowe.com.au/blog/item/24-what-we-all-should-know-about-depression.
76. www.theguardian.com/lifeandstyle/2010/aug/02/depression-mental-health-breakdown

77. https://cariadlloyd.com/griefcast
78. David Perlmutter and Austin Permutter. *Brain Wash*. 2020. London: Little Brown.
79. Adapted from Dr Daniel Amen.
80. www.nia.nih.gov/news/large-study-links-gum-disease-dementia
81. Rahul Jandial. *Life Lessons from a Brain Surgeon: The New Science and Stories of the Brain*. 2019. London: Penguin Life.
82. Oliver Scott Curry, Lee A. Rowland, Caspar J. Van Lissa, Sally Zlotowitz, John McAlaney, and Harvey Whitehouse. (2017) 'Happy to help? A systematic review and meta-analysis of the effects of performing acts of kindness on the well-being of the actor'. *Journal of Experimental Social Psychology*, 76.
83. S. Park, T. Kahnt, A. Doganet al. (2017) 'A neural link between generosity and happiness'. *Nature Communications*, 8: 15964. https://doi.org/10.1038/ncomms15964
84. www.theguardian.com/lifeandstyle/2023/jan/03/52-acts-of-kindness-how-to-spread-joy-in-every-week-of-2023?CMP=share_btn_link
85. See E. Brooke. *Women Healers Through History*. 2019. London: Aeon Books.
86. Chattergee, Rangan. Podcast, 9 December 2020 – www.drchatterjee.com
87. Julianne Holt-Lunstad, Bert N. Uchino, Timothy W. Smith, and Angela Hicks. (2017) 'On the Importance of Relationship Quality: The Impact of Ambivalence in Friendships on Cardiovascular Functioning'. *Annals of Behavioural Medicine* 33.3: 278–290.
88. P.M. Murphy and G.A. Kupshik. *Loneliness, Stress and Well-Being: a Helper's Guide*. 1992. Routledge.
89. I have written this up at length in my book *Women Healers through History*. 1993 [2002]. London: Aeon Bookspp. 261–265.
90. See TED Talk, Compassion Matters, Dr Julian Abel, Holt-Lunstad, Julianne, Timothy B Smith, and J Bradley Layton. (2010) 'Social Relationships and Mortality Risk: a Meta-Analytic Review'. *PLoS medicine* 7.7: e1000316–e1000316. 148 studies (308,849 participants), the random effects weighted average effect size was OR = 1.50 (95% CI 1.42 to 1.59), indicating a 50% increased likelihood of survival for participants with stronger

social relationships. This finding remained consistent across age, sex, initial health status, cause of death, and follow-up period. Significant differences were found across the type of social measurement evaluated (p, 0.001); the association was strongest for complex measures of social integration (OR = 1.91; 95% CI 1.63 to 2.23) and lowest for binary indicators of residential status (living alone versus with others).

91. https://drchatterjee.com/the-healing-power-of-compassion-with-dr-julian-abel, 9 December 2020.

92. www.theguardian.com/lifeandstyle/2022/dec/11/a-new-start-after-60

93. C. Boyce. (2023). 'I've spent years studying happiness – here's what actually makes for a happier life'. *The Conversation*, 2023 – https://theconversation.com/ive-spent-years-studying-happiness-heres-what-actually-makes-for-a-happier-life-197580

94. Avni Bavishi, Martin D. Slade, and Becca R. Levy. (2016) 'A chapter a day: Association of book reading with longevity'. *Social Science & Medicine*, 164: 44–48. https://doi.org/10.1016/j.socscimed.2016.07.014.(www.sciencedirect.com/science/article/pii/S0277953616303689).

95. Bavishi, Avni et al. (1982) 'A chapter a day: Association of book reading with longevity.' *Social science & medicine* 164 (2016): 44–48. doi:10.1016/j.socscimed.2016.07.014

96. R. Restak. (2023) 'An 81-year-old brain doctor's 7 "hard rules" for keeping your memory "sharp as a whip"' – www.cnbc.com/2023/02/02/81-year-old-neuroscience-shares-brain-rules-that-keep-his-memory-sharp-as-a-whip.html

97. S.A. Mehr, M.M. Krasnow, G.A. Bryant, and E.H. Hagen. (2021) 'Origins of music in credible signalling'. *Behavioural and Brain Sciences*, 44 (e60): 23–39. https://doi.org/10.1017/S0140525X20000345

98. H. Poikonen, P. Toiviainen, and M. Tervaniemi. (2018) 'Naturalistic music and dance: Cortical phase synchrony in musicians and dancers'. *PLoS ONE*, 13 (4): e0196065. https://doi.org/10.1371/journal.pone.0196065

99. Maxine Campion and Liat Levita. (2014) 'Enhancing positive affect and divergent thinking abilities: Play some music and dance'. *The Journal of Positive Psychology*, 9.2: 137–145. https://doi.org/10.1080/17439760.2013.848376

100. Zhang, Li-Xue, Chang-Xing Li, Mohib Ullah Kakar, Muham-mad Sajjad Khan, Pei-Feng Wu, Rai Muhammad Amir, Dong-Fang Dai et al. (2021) 'Resveratrol (RV): A Pharmaco-logical Review and Call for Further Research'. *Biomedicine & Pharmacotherapy*, 143: 112164–112164.

101. Andrew Scholey and Lauren Owen. (2013) 'Effects of chocolate on cognitive function and mood: a systematic review'. *Nutrition Reviews*, 71 (10): 665–681. https://doi.org/10.1111/nure.12065

102. www.nutritionadvance.com/chlorogenic-acid-health-benefits/ citing https://pubs.rsc.org/en/content/articlehtml/2014/fo/c4fo00290c

103. I. Onakpoya, E. Spencer, M. Thompson et al. (2015) 'The effect of chlorogenic acid on blood pressure: a systematic review and meta-analysis of randomized clinical trials'. *J. Hum. Hyper-tens.*, 29: 77–81. https://doi.org/10.1038/jhh.2014.46 and www.nutritionadvance.com/chlorogenic-acid-health-benefits/

104. Laura Y. Zuñiga et al. (2017) 'Effect of Chlorogenic Acid Admin-istration on Glycemic Control, Insulin Secretion, and Insulin Sensitivity in Patients with Impaired Glucose Tolerance'. *Jour-nal of Medicinal Food*, 21.5: 469–473. https://doi.org/10.1089/jmf.2017.0110 https://pubmed.ncbi.nlm.nih.gov/29261010/

105. Aidilla Mubarak, Catherine P. Bondonno, Alex H. Liu, Michael J. Considine, Lisa Rich, Emilie Mas, Kevin D. Croft, and Jonathan M. Hodgson. (2012) 'Acute effects of chloro-genic acid on nitric oxide status, endothelial function, and blood pressure in healthy volunteers: A randomized trial'. *Journal of Agricultural and Food Chemistry*, 60 (36): 9130–9136. https://doi.org/10.1021/jf303440j https://pubs.acs.org/doi/abs/10.1021/jf303440j

106. https://intothewylde.com/tag/boomers/

107. www.prnewswire.co.uk/news-releases/over-60s-more-confident-about-sex-than-ever-before-according-to-new-replens-survey-874379948.html

108. www.intothewylde.com sells a natural lubricant.

109. Joanie Mercier, Mélanie Morin, Dina Zaki, Barbara Reichetzer, Marie-Claude Lemieux, Samir Khalifé, and

Chantale Dumoulin. (2019) 'Pelvic floor muscle training as a treatment for genitourinary syndrome of menopause: A single-arm feasibility study'. *Maturitas*, 125: 57–62, https://doi.org/10.1016/j.maturitas.2019.03.002 (www.sciencedirect.com/science/article/pii/S0378512218307448).

110. See K. Bishop *It's Your Power Portal: Take Control of your Vaginal Health with Herbal and Holistic Care*. 2022. London: Aeon Books, pp. 140, 152.

111. www.psychologytoday.com/us/blog/all-about-sex/201811/ embers-back-flames-the-erotic-power-sexual-novelty – M. Castleman. (2018) 'Embers back to Flames: The erotic power of sexual novelty'. *Psychology Today*, 15 November 2018. www.psychologytoday.com/us/blog/all-about-sex/201811/ embers-back-flames-the-erotic-power-sexual-novelty

112. Bianca P. Acevedo, Arthur Aron, Helen E. Fisher, and Lucy L. Brown. (2012) 'Neural correlates of long-term intense romantic love'. *Social Cognitive and Affective Neuroscience*, 7.2: 145–159. https://doi-org.libezproxy.open.ac.uk/10.1093/scan/nsq092

113. Bianca P. Acevedo, Arthur Aron, Helen E. Fisher, and Lucy L. Brown. (2012) 'Neural correlates of long-term intense romantic love'. *Social Cognitive and Affective Neuroscience*, 7 (2): 145–159. https://doi-org.libezproxy.open.ac.uk/10.1093/scan/nsq092

114. www.traceycox.com/sex-conversation-starters/

115. www.sciencedirect.com/science/article/abs/pii/ S1047279713000914 Peter Muennig, Zohn Gretchen Johnson Rosen. (2013) 'Do the psychosocial risks associated with television viewing increase mortality? Evidence from the 2008 General Social Survey–National Death Index dataset'. *Annals of Epidemiology*, 23.6: 355–360. https://doi.org/10.1016/j.annepidem.2013.03.014

116. Dr Rangan Chatterjee. *This is the Most Powerful Tool to Improve your Health*. Podcast, December 2021. YouTube – www.youtube.com/watch?v=CUHYmbfHEVw&list=PLwAWbIQiqJ 0D2gn5UJBPSOzvLROyqSl7f

117. Adapted from Bonnie Ware. *The Top Five Regrets of the Dying*. 2019. London: Hay House.

118. See E. Brooke. *Women Healers Through History*. 2019. London: Aeon Books.
119. https://deathcafe.com/profile/49/
120. https://deathcafe.com/profile/61/
121. www.facebook.com/deathcafe
122. www.dignityindying.org.uk
123. www.dignityindying.org.uk/why-we-need-change/the-facts/
124. https://compassionindying.org.uk/
125. Felicity Warner. *A Safe Journey Home*. 2011. London: Hay House, p. 3.
126. Felicity Warner. *A Safe Journey Home*. 2011. London: Hay House, p. 13.
127. Felicity Warner. *A Safe Journey Home*. 2011. London: Hay House, p. 37.
128. Felicity Warner. *A Safe Journey Home*. 2011. London: Hay House, p. 38.
129. Felicity Warner. *A Safe Journey Home*. 2011. London: Hay House, p. 19.
130. Felicity Warner. *A Safe Journey Home*. 2011. London: Hay House, p. 32.
131. Felicity Warner. *A Safe Journey Home*. 2011. London: Hay House, p.80.
132. Felicity Warner. *Sacred Oils*. 2022. London: Hay House.
133. Felicity Warner. *A Safe Journey Home*. 2011. London: Hay House, p. 93.
134. Felicity Warner. *A Safe Journey Home*. 2011. London: Hay House, pp. 122–129.
135. Felicity Warner. *A Safe Journey Home*. 2011. London: Hay House, p. 192.
136. Felicity Warner. *A Safe Journey Home*. 2011. London: Hay House, p. 161.
137. Felicity Warner. *A Safe Journey Home*. 2011. London: Hay House, p. 113.
138. Felicity Warner. *A Safe Journey Home*. 2011. London: Hay House, p. 201.

139. Raymond A. Moody. (2013) 'Getting comfortable with death & near-death experiences. Near-death experiences: an essay in medicine & philosophy'. *Missouri Medicine*, 110.5: 368–371.

140. Raymond A. Moody. 'Getting comfortable with death & near-death experiences. Near-death experiences: an essay in medicine & philosophy'. *Missouri Medicine*, 110.5: 368–371.

141. Muslinclothsforjammakingworkwell,theycanbeboughtinJohn Lewis, Robert Dyas, or other kitchenware shops – www.robert-dyas.co.uk/kilner-muslin-square?_br_psugg_q=muslin+cloth

142. See Lucy Jones' book for more specific recipes and growing herbs.

143. https://tinandthyme.uk/2020/06/elderflower-champagne/

144. I go into greater detail about the herbs in my books, A Woman's Herbal and Traditional Western Herbal Medicine.

145. www.sciencedirect.com/topics/agricultural-and-biological-sciences/garlic

146. for more information see: https://draxe.com/nutrition/reishi-mushroom/

147. https://joinzoe.com/post/tim-spector-gut-tips

148. https://purehealthclinic.co.uk/2022/04/13/2022s-pesticide-fruit-and-veg-dirty-dozen-and-clean-fifteen/

149. www.niehs.nih.gov/health/materials/endocrine_disruptors_508.pdf#:~:text=Endocrine%20disruptors%20are%20found%20in%20everyday

150. www.thefiltery.com/volatile-organic-compounds-vocs-list/

151. A. Fleming. (2023) 'The Stress Secret: How to Meditate without Meditating'. *The Guardian*, 23 February 2023 – www.theguardian.com/lifeandstyle/2023/feb/09/the-stress-secret-12-ways-to-meditate-without-actually-meditating.

152. www.aeonbooks.co.uk/product/rest-is-radical-a-guide-to-deep-relaxation-through-yoga/94623/

INDEX

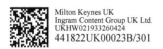
Milton Keynes UK
Ingram Content Group UK Ltd.
UKHW021933260424
441822UK00023B/301